The Challenge of Administering Health Services: Career Pathways

Edited by
Lowell Eliezer Bellin, M.D., M.P.H. and Lewis E. Weeks, Ph.D.
with the assistance of Marcia S. Lane

AUPHA PRESS
Washington, D.C.

TABLE OF CONTENTS

Preface

The sequence of jobs in the career odyssey of the flesh and blood health adminis-trator probably owes less to deliberate strategy than to fortuitous happenstance. The health administrator may spend the bulk of a career in one or more posts in any one of the individual specialties categorized separately in each of the chapters of this book. Or, the health administrator may switch specialties altogether, transferring from one to another that has apparently superior intellectual, political, spiritual, or financial allure.

No two health administrators' *curricula vitae* are the same. This book introduces the interested reader to some selected specialties in health administration. Most lay people are aware that health commissioners and hospital administrators exist. Yet, it has not occurred to them that hospital administrators and health commissioners be-long generically to a single professional discipline encompassing many other special-ties as well. Lay people know astonishingly little about the indispensable professional activities of those who manage and plan the health industry, with its enormous expenditure, payroll, and complexity, even though it so intimately impinges upon their very existence.

This book is not another textbook of health administration, although the reader ought to come away with a pretty good notion of what health administration is all about. Rather, the book consists of a series of chapters, each written by an expert in a health administration specialty. Space limitations obviously prevent the inclusion of health administrator types other than the most common and the most representative. In keeping with modern managerial style, contributing authors were not called upon to adhere to a single Procrustean outline. Variety supplanted uniformity. Individual proclivities determined what topics would receive emphasis, and in what order. The authors were encouraged to present vignettes or brief case studies and to be deliber-ately biographical in narrating what, why, and how they did things. The major proviso was that they avoid producing boredom.

Longevity and alleviation of biological and psychic misery are supposed to be the end products of health administration. A field professing such outcomes ought to have just claim on people of intellectual and moral excellence. The authors will deem their contributions successful if the book turns out to be a seductive recruiting device for the most talented, most socially dedicated, and most compassionate future colleagues available for health administration.

Lowell Eliezer Bellin, M.D., M.P.H.
New York City
March 10, 1980

Varieties of Health Administrator Education

Gary L. Filerman, Ph.D.

In health care the doctor-patient relationship has been supplemented, though not yet totally supplanted, by the organization-patient relationship. Managers run and control bureaucracies with varying success. In health care institutions, how well managers manage has survival implications for those service consumers called patients. People must be trained and socialized for their work roles, and health administrators are no exception to this rule. It is logical, then, to start this book with an analysis of the facts and the folklore of the education of health administrators. Although such education is taking place in various academic locations with diverse curricular philosophies, the alert reader will discern that certain principles are held in common and that educational convergence appears to be underway.

Gary L. Filerman, Ph.D., Executive Secretary of the recognized accrediting agency for education in health administration, the Accrediting Commission on Education for Health Services Administration (ACEHSA) presents an updated overview of the subject. (L.E.B.)

Introduction

The ensuing chapters of this book relate what health administrators do and where in the community they practice their profession. This chapter tells how to become a professional health administrator.

Health administration, often called health services administration, is a well-established and recognized profession. The numerous titles reflecting where administrators work and their special interests and training are all part of the same profession that works for the identical objective of managing the system that delivers health services to the public. Some of the most commonly used titles and specialties include: hospital administrator, health planner, nursing home administrator, clinic manager, health services administrator, and medical care administrator.

Health administrators belong to one or more professional associations. The largest of these is the American College of Hospital Administrators. Others include the American College of Nursing Home Administrators, the American College of Medical Group Administrators, the Canadian College of Health Service Executives, the American Health Planning Association, several sections of the American Public Health Association, the Association of Mental Health Administrators, and the National Association of Health Services Executives.

The master's degree in health administration is the most widely recognized professional preparation for a career in health administration. Only during the past twenty years has the master's degree gained the wide recognition it currently enjoys. Although there are still many top administrators who have other credentials, their num-

Gary L. Filerman, Ph.D., is Executive Secretary of the Accrediting Commission on Education for Health Services Administration. He is also President of the Association of University Programs in Health Administration (AUPHA).

ber is rapidly diminishing. It is prudent, therefore, for the ambitious newcomer to the field to earn a master's degree in administration from an accredited graduate program. The student can also earn a bachelor's degree in health administration, focusing on entry level preparation for those not immediately pursuing graduate study.

Employers such as public agencies, nonprofit boards of trustees, and nonprofit corporations, have come to look to professional health administrators for competent management. Health services have been called the most difficult management assignment in modern socie⁺y.

Professional education and practice in health administration bring together the knowledge and skills of many disciplines. Health administration, then, is not a single discipline like economics, political science, or sociology. Health administration builds upon such disciplines and others, including medicine, engineering, epidemiology, organizational behavior, accounting, financial management, and statistics.

In recent years research has provided insight into what contributes to or detracts from high quality health service. Sophisticated and expensive technology is often falsely believed to ensure high quality, as are the elaborate credentials of physicians and other practitioners. Neither do large, modern, and antiseptic looking hospitals and clinics automatically generate high quality. In fact, quality may be defined by the attention given to prevention, by the use of less complicated treatment, and by services other than those normally considered part of medical treatment, such as good advice about daily living and assistance with family responsibilities. Within the medical setting, quality frequently depends upon each health worker's willingness to go beyond the limitations of the technical job. Such a spirit, which can be found in a poorly equipped rural health clinic as well as in a great city hospital, is the result of leadership. Leadership is the major ingredient that the health administrator is supposed to contribute to the system.

Careers in health services administration are not closed to those without the master's degree in health administration. Many individuals lacking the degree but located in key health services administration roles have been trained in medicine, nursing, business administration, public administration, etc. However, as mentioned, their number is diminishing while the number of professional health services administrators is growing. Not surprisingly, many such individuals entered the field decades ago before health administration became so complex as to require special preparation.

Types of Programs

The Bachelor's Degree

Undergraduate degrees in health administration are a new development. Substantial programs with full-time, well-trained, and experienced faculty have been operating only since the early seventies. Many less well-developed undergraduate programs may consist of a single full-time faculty member or may be organized around part-time faculty who are practicing health administrators. The newness and variety of the undergraduate degrees make it difficult to generalize about what such a degree will mean professionally in years to come. The number of graduates is small, and they have been in the field for too brief a time for us to draw valid conclusions as yet about what kind of positions bachelor's degree holders will eventually hold.

Some undergraduate programs offer fine educations while others offer limited instruction. Many bachelor's degree holders have launched successful careers while others feel that they lack access to positions they prefer. Clearly, the prospective student should investigate undergraduate programs carefully to determine the quality of the background and access to the field the program will provide. At present, no accreditation mechanism exists specifically for undergraduate programs in health administration.

What kind of preparation do the undergraduate programs provide? Some programs define objectives identical to those of graduate programs: to prepare the enrollee

2

for senior administrative responsibilities in the largest and most complex health organizations. These programs focus upon community hospitals, health planning agencies, ambulatory care programs, regulatory agencies, and insurance programs. Some of the graduates with bachelor's degrees are competing successfully with holders of master's degrees for these positions and will undoubtedly capture some of the most challenging of them as they have the opportunity to demonstrate their abilities.

Most undergraduate programs focus upon the top management of less complex organizations and upon the middle management of the large organizations. The latter include some of the most important unmet management needs in the field. Excellent opportunities exist here for competent holders of bachelor's degrees. In fact, some observers believe that the solid grounding in a specialized field of middle management provided by a bachelor's degree education gives strong competitive advantage to the specialist over the generalist.

Bachelor's degree programs concentrate upon management opportunities in nursing homes, group medical practices, and unit management in hospitals. Unit managers coordinate all of the services and personnel of a hospital nursing unit. They also prepare department heads for complex management assignments such as hospital central services, materials management, purchasing, security, admissions, and the business office. In some very large hospitals, each of these functions involves more personnel and a bigger budget than the entire hospital of average size.

A third group of undergraduate programs is more specialized, concentrating on preparation for the hospital's business office, hospital accounting, or health financial management. The degree is usually a Bachelor of Business Administration with a concentration in health finance, for example. Most of the courses duplicate those taken by all B.B.A. candidates, with an added sequence of courses applied to health organizations.

Admission to a bachelor's program usually occurs at the beginning of the junior year. At that point the student can transfer most readily into one of the programs within the college or university or to another school. Since transfer into a program becomes more difficult thereafter, the student should decide on an undergraduate health administration degree during the freshman or sophomore year.

However, an undergraduate health administration degree is not strictly recommended as preparation for a graduate degree in the field. Graduates of bachelor programs have been admitted to some graduate programs, but there is no evidence of a competitive advantage for admission. In fact, many graduate programs prefer students who have completed a strong general education program rather than one designed to equip them to enter the profession at the bachelor's level. As undergraduate programs develop and graduates demonstrate their potential, this situation will most likely change.

The Master's Degree

Master's degree programs in health administration differ. The programs themselves have various titles, such as health administration, health care administration, health services management, medical care organization, hospital administration, health planning, and a number of combinations of these basic terms. To complicate the situation further, accredited health administration programs offer about a dozen different degrees. In order of frequency earned, they include:

- Master of Health/Health Services Administration
- Master in Business Administration (in health administration)
- Master of Public Administration
- Master of Science in Hospital/Hospital and Health Services/Health Care Administration
- Master in Hospital Administration
- Master of Arts in Health/Hospital/Hospital and Health Services/Health Care Administration

3

- Master of Public Health
- Master of Management in Hospital and Health Services Administration

All accredited graduate programs require two years of full-time study or the equivalent. The programs may include up to one year spent as an administrative resident in a health program or facility. Post-graduate residencies/fellowships are also increasingly being offered to students as complements to graduate training.

Substantial differences exist between schools' emphasis on required topics and content. Students enrolled in a program in a business school may take courses required by all M.B.A. students. The same is true of programs in public health (the M.P.H.) or public administration (the M.P.A.). These differences give the potential student the opportunity to pick a program that builds upon his or her previous undergraduate or professional background.

The public benefits from this flexibility, as it ensures that all health services administrators will not analyze problems in the same way. Complex health administration problems require creative thinking and a variety of skills and perspectives. When the people tackling problems bring diverse approaches to bear on them, they increase the likelihood of an imaginative solution in the public interest. This diversity by design continues to be nurtured by the leadership of health administration despite the problems created by the absence of a commonly labeled academic degree.

Factors to Consider in Choosing a Program

Acknowledging this diversity, what should a prospective health administrator look for in a graduate program? One consideration is accreditation. A program may be subject to or influenced by up to three academic accreditations. The first is the college's or university's basic accreditation. It is called "regional" accreditation because it is carried out by one of several regional associations of colleges and universities across the United States. Regional accreditation applies to the total institution, its administration, resources, administrative practices, and major teaching activities, ensuring that all institutions provide a basic level of educational quality. A number of institutions offering education for various health disciplines are not regionally accredited.

The other two types of accreditation, variations of the same system, are called programmatic accreditation. This type of accreditation focuses on specific programs or professions, and is carried out by associations of professional schools, organizations of professionals, or commissions combining such interests. While programmatic accreditation operates in many professional fields, there are many more in which it does not. In part, the variation affecting health services administration results from the fact that many of the graduate programs belong to or are affiliated with larger schools that are programmatically accredited for other purposes. The two most frequent examples are the programs related to accredited schools of business administration and accredited schools of public health. There are also programs related to accredited schools of pharmacy and medicine. Many programs are related to schools of public administration, allied health or graduate schools, for which there is no programmatic accreditation.

Graduate programs in health administration are accredited by an agency organized specifically for this field. Accreditation by the Accrediting Commission on Education for Health Services Administration (ACEHSA) is the most important assurance to the potential student that a program meets the minimum criteria developed by the profession and the health services system. The Accrediting Commission is the only agency recognized for this purpose by the Council on Postsecondary Accreditation (COPA), which regulates accreditation on behalf of the nation's colleges, universities, and the public.

The ACEHSA is cosponsored by the major organizations in the field, the American College of Hospital Administrators, American College of Nursing Home Administrators, American College of Medical Group Administrators, American Public Health

4

Association, American Hospital Association, and the Association of University Programs in Health Administration. There are also two consulting members: Association of Mental Health Administrators and the American Health Planning Association. Accreditation by ACEHSA carries the influence of approval by the principal employers and peers of program graduates.

Some other factors should be considered. New programs are not eligible for accreditation until they have actually awarded degrees; therefore, programs less than two years old cannot be accredited. It is helpful to know, therefore, whether a program is or is not preparing for accreditation. Programs are accredited for various periods up to five years, but a shorter accreditation does not mean that the program is inferior. Rather, it means that the Commission monitors progress and development over short periods to assure the public and the profession that existing and potential problems are being considered.

Individuals who are interested in learning more about accreditation can write directly to the Commission for a list of accredited graduate programs, for a list of dates when the programs will be reviewed, and for a copy of the criteria used for accreditation. The address is:

Accrediting Commission on Education
for Health Services Administration
One Dupont Circle—Suite 420
Washington, D.C. 20036

Another indication of quality is membership in the Association of University Programs in Health Administration (AUPHA). AUPHA requires that its member programs either be accredited or be working toward accreditation. A list of members is available from the Association at the following address:

Office of Research and Student Affairs
AUPHA
1755 Massachusetts Ave., N.W.—Suite 310
Washington, D.C. 20036

Accreditation is not as widely used in Canada as it is in the United States. No voluntary regional accreditation of the total college or university exists, but provincial agencies monitor basic quality. Canadian graduate programs in health services administration do, however, participate fully in the Accrediting Commission on Education for Health Services Administration. Canadian educators were instrumental in the Commission's formation, and Canadians occasionally serve on the Commission. Education in health administration in the two nations is closely associated, with students and faculty frequently moving between the two. Canadian and American degrees are reciprocally recognized, and Canadian programs fully participate in AUPHA.

The health administration program's quality usually exists independently of the university or the school of which it is a part. Excellent programs exist in relatively unknown universities. The opposite is also true: some programs with inadequate resources may be found in well-known universities. Therefore, it is imperative to investigate programs rather than universities.

The potential applicant can learn much about a program by reading and comparing catalogs from several programs, by talking to alumni and students, and by visiting the program. When applying, it is appropriate to ask for the names of alumni and students with whom one can visit. If the program requires an interview for admission, the applicant can convert the visit into a two-way exploration. Two years, after all, is an expensive once-in-a-lifetime investment. The applicant need not hesitate to interview faculty just as faculty interviews the student. Even if the program does not require an interview, it is wise to ask for one. An interview will not only provide useful background but also probably enhance chances of gaining admission.

What should the applicant look for? First, a challenging environment, one that encourages the student to probe deeply into the subjects covered and the issues of the

5

day. Evidence of this desirable characteristic is close contact with the faculty, both in seminars and through supervision of written work and other projects. The conscientious student wants no less than a rigorous gradute program encouraging the type of thorough analysis that will be expected of the professional in the field. Are the faculty members well-known as writers and consultants actually working with and available to the students? Have faculty members achieved the university's senior rank that often measures scholarship? Do faculty members conduct research and publish? What are the research interests of program faculty?

The scope of the program is important. In addition to professional education, ask whether faculty conduct doctoral level education—a good indicator of an intellectually active environment. Participation by faculty in continuing education of practicing health service administrators indicates academic immersion in real world problems. But the most important determinant of the program's scope can be measured by what the program hopes its graduates will contribute, what they will be doing in their careers.

Programs' objectives also differ. Some concentrate on the senior administrative role in general acute hospitals. Others concentrate upon communitywide health services planning. Others try to avoid such specificity in order to provide the broadest possible overview of the total system. Some programs offer the opportunity to select tracks that may consist of several courses in such functional specialties as health planning, policy analysis, or the administration of health maintenance organizations, general hospitals, ambulatory care, long-term care, or mental health programs.

Educational philosophy will determine whether a program's curriculum should prepare every graduate for a top-level administrative assignment or for a first, lower-level job.

Beyond a certain minimum, the size of a program faculty alone is not a good measure of quality for the potential student. A program with only two or three full-time faculty probably cannot effectively meet student needs. On the other hand, a large faculty can mean good resources, but it can also mean that the program does not take advantage of the resources of the rest of the university. The applicant is advised to investigate the implications of minimal faculty size only, keeping in mind that there are exceptional cases of small faculties well supported by their school's entire faculty.

However, this raises an interesting question about how to use the university. Health services administration must draw upon the knowledge and skills of many disciplines in order to understand and cope with the complex problem of health services delivery. How great is the student's access to those disciplines? No program possesses all the resources necessary to fulfill all academic requirements through its own faculty. Are there opportunities to take courses in fields in which the student may develop a special interest, even if the courses are offered in another part of the university? The student may have a good background in one or more of the key content areas before beginning the program. Many programs offer opportunities to select electives, but the actual freedom of choice differs substantially among the schools. Some programs do not offer any or many electives because of the heavy demands of the core content in health services administration and/or the requirements of the core curriculum for the degree. The latter is particularly characteristic of the M.B.A. and M.P.H. Looking into this question will provide insight into the program's organization, resources, and educational philosophy.

Most health administration educators and practitioners agree that both undergraduate and graduate programs ought to include a substantial experience in the real world. A period of work in any actual health program or facility helps the student grasp the relevance of course work. As a result, almost every program has a field experience component; however, programs differ markedly in the way they handle this portion of the curriculum.

The term residency is widely used to describe the most substantial field work component, and the student carries the title administrative resident while completing the residency requirement. Residencies required for the degree may be as short as three months (the summer between two academic years) or as long as twelve months. Some graduate programs consist of one academic year of eight or nine months and a twelve-month residency in a health program or facility. Others require three semesters of course work and five or six months' residency. There are other patterns as well.

Most programs requiring the residency also require the students to be enrolled and to pay tuition for its duration. At the same time the student generally receives a stipend from the residency health institution or program while working there. Most programs require all students in residency to spend the period doing similar activities, although they may be scattered across the country in different kinds of health service organizations. The residency is a period of on-the-job observation and study. It is not to be viewed as low-paid work.

Most programs have close ties with a few well-chosen administrators of health services delivery organizations with whom the students spend the residency periods. These administrators are called preceptors and may actually have appointments as adjunct members of the university faculties. They are selected for their demonstrated professional leadership and interest in education. The student studies the preceptor as well as the health program. Preceptor selection and supervision of the residency are a measure of graduate program quality. Students with limited knowledge of the field should not make their own residency arrangements. It is very important to look for programs that treat the residency, whatever its length, as an integral part of the program and pay close attention to the quality of the student experience.

An increasing number of programs do not require a residency on the premise that the student may not study formally after entering the field and should, therefore, devote all of his or her time to formal class work. This approach assumes that the graduate will have many opportunities to learn about the world of work and to progress gradually through management development. Such programs usually include field work without large time commitments.

The academic programs (to distinguish them from the residency programs) may strongly encourage students to work in the health field during the summers. This is particularly true when the student has no previous health experience. Some programs include close continuing relationships with selected health organizations that offer first jobs resembling residencies. These are management-development positions tailored to the needs of the individual and without formal ties to the university.

No evidence suggests that graduates of one or the other type of program are more successful or qualified; however, a clear preference is growing for the two-year academic model, with or without the summer field work requirement. Health services organizations are rapidly changing from independent hospitals, nursing homes, and health centers to large systems of units of different kinds or all hospitals. These multipurpose or multihospital systems present an ideal environment for a management development experience based upon a two-year academic program.

Applying for Admission

The most important point to consider when making application plans is that the competition differs significantly among the programs. Some accredited programs accept fewer than 20 students a year and others accept 50 or more. Some of the older, better known programs receive twelve or fourteen applications for each place. Some of the lesser known programs have an acceptance ratio of two to one. Obviously, an applicant with a reasonably good record may not get into one program while easily gaining admission to another. You'll never know if you don't apply.

Every year excellent applicants are turned away because they failed to follow the most sagacious application strategy. The first step of this strategy is to begin early. The applicant should write for catalogs and become familiar with the programs a full year before application. It is wise to start in the fall of the senior year of college, since

7

applications should be submitted in January of the year in which the applicant hopes to enter. By December of the year before the program starts, the applicant should have completed application plans, having made at least first, second, and third choices. The most selective programs will have filled their classes by February or March for the following fall. Some programs admit a very few students in midyear, and most admit students only in the fall.

No strategy will work without the appropriate foundation. The building blocks of that foundation are the undergraduate academic record, undergraduate majors, scores on standard tests, work experience, recommendations, demonstrated leadership ability, and prerequisite courses. The earlier in the academic career the applicant starts preparing for graduate school, the more likely he or she is to have all of the right building blocks, and to gain admission to the program of choice. Of course, there is no guarantee. Different programs look for different things. The student who investigates the programs thoroughly knows that.

The most commonly used criterion for admission to a graduate program is undergraduate grade point average. Clearly, most faculty members, despite questioning the relevance of grades as a predictor of professional success, continue to look at grades first. Grades remain a major consideration when an applicant has been out of school for several years. Grades reflect self-discipline and may relate to one's ability to handle some of the challenging quantitative content that is essential for modern health services administration.

Undergraduate major or previous professional education is also important, and is considered quite differently among the programs. The value of an undergraduate major in health services administration was discussed earlier. Overall, undergraduate liberal arts majors prevail among successful applicants, with business majors the next highest. Faculties seem to prefer the students with the broadest possible educational backgrounds. The program is less likely to have to repeat introductory material on the social sciences for such students. The business undergraduate is most likely to have required background for admission to the programs affiliated with business schools and awarding the M.B.A. degree in health administration.

Regardless of the undergraduate major, many programs favor strong quantitative content. Quantitative content can be gained in calculus, statistics, advanced mathematics, operations research, finance, economics, psychology, and other areas. The strong trend toward increased quantitative content in the graduate program assumes that quantitative skills will be required for effective administration of health services in the future.

Previous training in another health field such as medicine, dentistry, nursing, and planning, or in a profession such as law or social work, is no guarantee for gaining admission to a graduate program. Studies for such professions often do not include adequate preparation in such key areas as quantitative skills. It is recommended that individuals with previous professional training obtain the advice of program faculty before applying.

Unlike some other fields, in health administration there is no single standard test that is used by all programs. Although not all programs require tests, all pay attention to available scores, especially when the grade point average is a source of doubt. The most frequently used tests are the Graduate Record Examination (GRE)-Aptitude, Graduate Management Admission Test (GMAT) and Miller Analogies Test (MAT). Although there is controversy over whether the tests accurately predict academic performance, a good score definitely impresses most admission committees. Most large colleges and universities have testing centers where anyone can take such examinations. However, some are administered only on certain dates that can be months away; so it is incumbent upon the potential applicant to start early.

Programs take previous health-related work experience into consideration, although few formally require this for admission. Previous experience shows motivation and provides contacts who are fruitful sources of recommendations for the graduate programs. Useful experience is hard to define, but three schools of thought exist on the subject among faculty. One group would say that the prospective administrator should get as close to administration as possible. That would mean part-time and summer work in a hospital admitting office, the business office of a neighborhood health center, or a similar job. Another faculty group would say that any job in the health setting would give insight into the way the system works. These jobs might include ambulance attendant, file clerk in a group practice, or computer programmer in a health planning agency.The third view argues that contact with the community served is the most critical experience, because administrators frequently lack insight into the needs of the people served by the system. These jobs would include hospital orderlies or receptionists at outpatient clinics and health maintenance organizations, where the employee's public contact would be valued more highly than the content of his or her job. Given this interest in experience, it is valuable to get some, part-time or summer, but not at the expense of grades. It is also true that some applicants who do not gain admission to a program one year are successful after a year of experience in a health service organization.

Developing some relevant experience also leads to familiarity with people in the field. As mentioned, these are ideal sources of recommendations when it comes time to apply. Managers who have observed the applicant working with others in an organization have more impact than the family clergyman or physician. Applicants should be aware that a tradition exists—most clearly in general hospitals—by which administrators take special interest in individuals aspiring to enter health administration programs. That interest is often expressed by finding the student a job where he or she can see more of the total institution or program or by inviting the student to meetings and other events of interest. This recognition can only take place if the student makes his or her long-range goals known to the senior administrator. We therefore suggest that the student do so.

In a highly competitive situation program faculties will seek distinctive characteristics that appear to correlate with success in the field. Leadership is one such characteristic. Leadership can be a record of activity in religious youth groups, student government, campus political clubs, student journalism, and service organizations. These activities stimulate creativity, provide valuable human relations and political skills, and show breadth of interest. Nevertheless, it deserves repeating that student involvement is inadequate justification for poor academic performance.

The final foundation blocks are the prerequisite courses, that is, the courses that the student must complete before beginning the graduate program. Not all programs have prerequisite courses. Others will admit a student on the condition that they be completed before the program starts—usually the preceding summer. In a few cases missing prerequisites can be taken along with the program during the first quarter or semester.

There are three reasons for prerequisites. First, they reduce the need to teach undergraduate material at the graduate level. It is still necessary to cover a great deal of introductory content that differs little from that included in earlier stages of education. Secondly, the prerequisites ensure a certain degree of common ground in the class. Through them, everyone, regardless of background, builds the same base in at least some key areas. Third, an applicant's performance in a key course such as calculus or economics may show aptitude in a subject essential to successfully completing the program.

The most frequently required prerequisite is accounting, and every future administrator is well advised to have an introductory course at the undergraduate level. The material taught in a full semester or more at the undergraduate level is usually reviewed in the first three weeks of a graduate program; therefore, it is wise to have learned its basic principles. Economics is also favored as a prerequisite, for both the analytic experience and the basic knowledge it provides are a base upon which the student can build a knowledge of health economics. Some programs will require at least one course in a biological science as an introduction to scientific thought. Other prerequisites include quantitative methods, statistics, measurement, mathematics or a behavioral science (usually psychology and/or sociology). Most graduate programs require from zero to three prerequisites, but some M.B.A.-based programs practically insist on a B.B.A. or close to it for admission.

After identifying the programs of greatest interest, a wise strategy is to apply early to all of them and to take seriously each of their requirements and suggestions. As mentioned, if the program suggests but does not require an interview with an alumnus, arrange for the interview. It does not make good sense to apply to one or two programs and to wait to hear from them before applying to some of the newer, lesser known programs, some of which are among the strongest.

The selective programs are not all looking for the same characteristics. Of course, as a minimum, all look for solid evidence of ability to perform graduate work, but when 100 good people apply for 25 places, other factors come into play. A common one is mix, based upon the assumption that students learn from each other and that different student backgrounds make for an exciting learning environment. Thus, an admission committee may look for some students with experience and other without, given a minimal grade point average.

Financial Aid

Health services administration education, like all graduate education, is expensive. Student aid is available at most programs, either from government or private sources. In spite of the problems it causes, putting together an effective student assistance "package" almost always depends upon gaining admission first. If a candidate is very strong, some programs may offer assurances of financial aid at the time of application, but this is unusual. In the United States, the insecurity involved in seeking financial aid is exacerbated when universities are not informed of the amount of federal aid they will receive until late spring, long after classes have been notified of admission.

The most common form of federal aid in the U.S. is the traineeship, which pays tuition and some other expenses. In Canada, similar assistance comes in the form of bursaries from some provincial governments. Some programs have loan funds contributed by alumni. Both Canadian and U.S. accredited programs have Foster McGaw scholarships, both of which are administered by the Association of University Programs in Health Administration (AUPHA). In addition, both the American College of Hospital Administrators and AUPHA maintain loan funds for minority students. Access to these resources is available only through the faculty of the program to which you are admitted. Information about the financial aid available at a specific university may be obtained by writing to the program director and the financial aid officer.

A summer work-study program for the purpose of acquainting interested minority group undergraduates with the field of health services administration is sponsored jointly by AUPHA and the National Association of Health Services Executives. This program enables talented sophomore and junior students to spend a summer working and studying in a hospital or other health care organization. During 1980, over 85 minority group students in 10 cities across the country participated in this work-study program. Inquiries regarding application materials should be directed to: The Office of Educational Opportunity, AUPHA, 1755 Massachusetts Avenue, N.W.—Suite 308, Washington, D.C. 20036.

Professional Placement

It may appear premature to think about placement in a starting position while still in the application stage. However, differences in placement systems and patterns distinguish one program from another. Health administration has two distinct job placement systems. One is an open system much like those in other fields. The program helps the student get started if it can, but the fledgling professional is really

10

on his or her own. The potential graduate makes use of contacts already developed, places ads, responds to ads, and visits health services organizations.

In the other more directed system, the program faculty takes a direct hand in initial placement. Alumni are expected to inform the program before anyone else when they know of positions opening up. Some of these programs have well-organized systems that function almost like commercial placement firms. One of the weaknesses of these systems is that they usually do little placement outside hospitals. Of course, being a part of these alumni systems does not preclude the use of other approaches to finding a position in an organization that seems attractive.

Outlook

The outlook for graduates of a good program is bright. The field of health administration is exapnding vertically and horizontally—vertically since large organizations are adding more program graduates to take on a wide variety of administrative responsibilities, and horizontally because the important contributions of professional health services administrators are being recognized by more and more organizations. New kinds of opportunities are opening up constantly for the dedicated and well-trained health administrator.

2   As Hospital Administrator

Raymond S. Alexander, M.B.A., M.H.A.

One of the most familiar specialties in health administration, of course, is hospital adminis-tration. The hospital administrator runs an institution that is often of incredible complexity and magnitude, has charge of a formidable budget, and oversees a perplexing assortment of profes-sionals, paraprofessionals, and other auxiliary personnel, who perform more than 100 separate jobs. The newer economic facts of life, particularly the increasingly scarce governmental sources of funding, and the dynamics of the consumer movement, have eroded the autonomy of hospitals. The hospital administrator must pay sober attention to the extramural forces that besiege the institution. Hospital structure, program, and administration will reflect, more and more, the imperatives of advancing technology and the simultaneous demands for economy.

Ray Alexander has spent most of his career in hospital administration. He shares his views in this chapter. (L.E.B.)

Historical Perspective

Phenomenal growth in hospitals has occurred over the last 100 years. In 1873, there were only 149 hospitals in the country, whose combined bed capacity was 35,453. Hospital growth mushroomed in the twentieth century, as did the population. In 1978 there were 7,015 hospitals with 1,381,000 beds. Experts attribute this astounding growth to three factors: the development of adjunct services, such as diagnostic and therapeutic services; the innovation and expansion of hospital insurance plans; and greater public confidence in hospital care. The image of the hospital as a place to die was displaced by that of a scientific institution for the diagnosis and treatment of illness. One can add to this list other factors, such as the advent of Medicare and Medicaid in 1965, enfranchising some 30,000,000 Americans for hospital services; the growing complexity of medical care, causing greater reliance by the physician on sophisticated hospital tests and procedures; and the movement to deinstitutionalize hospitals by providing high quality hotel services in attractive surroundings.

The hospital industry today accounts for over 40 percent of all the funds spent for health services in the United States. In 1978 this amounted to 70 billion dollars. In 1976, there were 4.5 hospital beds in community hospitals for every 1,000 people and, on the average, one out of six Americans was hospitalized in 1978.

As a consequence, the profession of hospital administration has undergone a concomitant growth, presently employing some 17,500 people in hospital managerial positions. Over 6,700 students are enrolled in the 67 graduate level American and Canadian programs of hospital and health administration belonging to the Association

Raymond S. Alexander, M.B.A., M.H.A., is President and Chief Executive Officer of the Albert Einstein Medical Center in Philadelphia, Pennsylvania. He is Adjunct Assistant Professor at the Columbia University School of Public Health and Administrative Medicine and is also Adjunct Professor of Health Care Systems at the Wharton School, University of Pennsylvania.

of University Programs in Health Administration (AUPHA). Each year 50 to 60 percent of the graduates find employment in positions classified as hospital administration. We shall examine the field of *hospital* administration as a subset of *health* administration.

Hospital Industry Today

The hospital industry today hardly resembles that of 50 years ago. The changes account in large measure for the growth of the field of hospital administration. The modern hospital performs a wide variety of functions, depending upon its size, location, community need, resources, leadership, and institutional philosophy and commitment. These functions can be summarized as follows:

1. *Service*—This function includes care to the patient and can encompass preventive, diagnostic, curative, and rehabilitative services on both an inpatient (hospitalized) and an outpatient (ambulatory) basis. The hospital provides the "gathering point" for the skilled personnel, specialized facilities, and appropriate machinery needed to perform these activities. The hospital embraces emergency room facilities, diagnostic x-ray rooms, surgical suites, and technologically advanced instruments to analyze blood, examine tissue, or irradiate tumors.
2. *Education*—This function covers a wide range of educational activities. Physicians in medical school, residents at a postgraduate level, nurses, medical technologists, radiologic technicians, and hospital administrators are types of students who may receive education in a hospital. In addition, continuing medical education occurs for physicians at a number of levels. Also, many institutions seek to educate their patients and the general public.
3. *Research*—Both applied and basic research can take place at the hospital, depending upon resources, medical school relationships, interests of the medical staff, and motivation.

The goals and objectives of some institutions include entering into a variety of social health programs such as neighborhood redevelopment, public health education, the operation of nursing homes and home health services, and satellite ambulatory care units. Other activities might include programs to generate additional sources of revenue, such as a physicians' office building, parking ramps, the sale of management services, and so on.

Hospitals today occupy a pivotal place in our society. Many health planners feel that future delivery systems will be centered around the hospital system with its assemblage of buildings, equipment, physician manpower, and management skills. A hospital can be a significant economic force in a community, often functioning as its major employer. Its impact can be extensive, drawing patients from surrounding communities, or even from other parts of the country.

A volume entitled *Hospital Statistics* contains more than 200 pages of data detailing the characteristics of today's hospitals. The current edition, published each year by the American Hospital Association (AHA), underscores the diversity and complexity of the field. In addition to the statistical guide, the AHA publishes yearly a *Guide to the Health Care Field*, listing, by geographic locations, AHA-registered and osteopathic hospitals in the United States and associated areas; U.S. government hospitals outside the United States; and accredited long-term care facilities.

Leafing through these two volumes, one begins to appreciate the industry's scope and complexity. Of the 7,156 hospitals, the majority (5,875) are community hospitals (nonfederal, whose facilities are available to the public) and short-term (patients stay fewer than 30 days). Most of the community hospitals (almost 80 percent) are under 200 beds in size, and very few (less than 5 percent) are over 500 beds. As in other industries, the smaller institutions are decreasing in number, while the larger ones increase in size.

Taking into consideration the federal hospital system, the state and local governmental hospitals, the investor-owned (for profit) hospitals, as well as the community

14

(not for profit) hospitals, one begins to comprehend the importance of management in a system this vast.

Evolution of Hospital Administration

As hospitals grew in size and influence in the twentieth century, it became clear that they needed to be directed by qualified individuals. As early as 1910 it was recognized that special training was required to run a hospital. In the early 1900s, the traditional manager was a nurse or a physician, referred to as superintendents. Training took place largely on the job, and those interested in a career were apprentices to the superintendent. It was not until 1929 that Michael Davis wrote what was to become a landmark in the field, a book entitled *Hospital Administration: A Career*. In 1932 his findings were further reinforced by the Committee on the Costs of Medical Care, which included, among other recommendations, that hospitals and clinics should be viewed as social and business enterprises as well as medical institutions, and that it was important that they be directed by trained administrators.

In 1934, the first course in hospital administration was established by Michael Davis at the University of Chicago in the Graduate School of Business. A Master of Business Administration degree was awarded after an academic year on campus and a twelve-month administrative residency in a selected hospital off campus. Subsequently, courses were started at Northwestern University in 1943, Columbia University in 1946, and the University of Toronto, the University of California, and Yale in 1947. Other schools were soon established in universities around the country. Once referred to as programs in hospital administration, these schools have recognized the changing nature of the field and have redesignated themselves programs in health administration or health services administration. As previously mentioned, the national association of these programs, formed in 1948, refers to itself as the AUPHA—the Association of University Programs in Health Administration (formerly Hospital Administration). In February 1981 AUPHA membership figures listed 97 graduate and undergraduate programs throughout the United States and Canada.

A number of commissions were formed over the past 30 years to examine the nature of this new profession and to determine what courses of instruction needed to be taught, how educational efforts could be upgraded, and how managerial effectiveness and performance could be improved. In 1945, a Joint Commission on Education examined the educational requirements for entry into hospital administration. Their studies revealed that when top jobs opened, hospital governing boards usually sought men with medical training, while boards of smaller institutions usually preferred a nurse. Through the efforts of this Commission, six new training centers came into being, and a core curriculum was described consisting of work in the following areas: the medical staff, personnel management, hospital departments and departmental functioning; medical care programs; business and financial management; and community relations.

In 1954, the Commission on University Education in Hospital Administration conducted a study of education for administrators of hospitals envisioned for the future and advanced recommendations for improvements of present programs. The Commission believed that a liberal arts education blended with certain basic courses in professional and functional fields of administration would be the best preparation. Foundation courses were considered to be mathematics and statistics, psychology, sociology, economics; functional fields were identified as finance, marketing, and personnel. The Commission felt that any plan of instruction should include five general objectives:

1. Knowledge of organization and management of hospitals.
2. Competence in the orderly exploration and solution of problems and decision making in the area of administration.
3. Effective dealing with people, both individually and in groups, and skill in communication.

4. Thorough understanding of the economic and social system in which we live and in which the hospital operates.
5. An inquiring mind, independence of thought, and maturity of character.

The Commission also set standards for the faculty, for the function of the school in a university setting, and for the program director's qualifications.

In 1974, a third study was completed under the auspices of the W.K. Kellogg Foundation. This study, which began in 1972, again addressed the status of health administrators' education and its relevance to contemporary health delivery problems. This study commission concerned itself with the proliferation of educational programs and their graduates; significant changes in basic curricula; growing interest in many universities in the development of undergraduate programs; and the relationship between hospital administration education and other parallel programs such as public health administration, medical care organization, and comprehensive health planning. The commission also examined the relationship between management and the provision of health services: namely, whether improved management makes an impact on the problems of access to health care, its comprehensiveness, cost, and continuity.

The commission's findings directly affected the future of health administration and are of great significance to the reader. In its report, *Education for Health Administration* (Vol. 1, p. 14), the Commission determined that:

1. Fewer than 25 percent of executive positions are filled by individuals with formal training in health administration. Therefore, a great deal more emphasis needs to be placed on educating new and current practitioners through a variety of strategies.
2. Lifelong learning opportunities need to be provided so as to ensure continuing competence for practicing administrators.
3. The educational content of programs must be improved to prepare administrators for leadership positions. Basic core curricula should consist of education in a) health, that is, information on health and disease, health and medical care organization, and environmental management; and b) administration, that is, theory and skills relating to social organization and the political process. There also needs to be more interaction between didactic work and field experience. To enhance the education of administrators, more specialist training in finance, personnel management, and system engineering should be encouraged.
4. Educational quality needs to be enhanced by increasing faculty size, program visibility, and relationships with health practice.
5. Student quality and recruitment need to be improved by expanding the pool of program applicants.
6. Interdependency in education should be stressed by collaborating with other disciplines such as medical education, social work, public administration, and law.

The Commission concluded by reiterating the importance of administration in the health and medical care system because of the following changes:

1. Strengthened state and areawide planning regulations.
2. Increased emphasis on the promotion of health.
3. Promotion of efficiency in delivery of services.
4. Promotion of public accountability.
5. Continuing research into planning, organization, and administration.
6. Establishment of effective social policy.

Many of the findings and recommendations of these studies have been incorporated into the curricula of the programs in health administration. Programs may be found in separate university departments, or in schools of business administration, public health, medicine, allied health, or other settings. For details, refer to chapter 1, Varieties of Health Administrator Education, by Gary L. Filerman.

What Do Administrators Do?

The changes in the educational process reflect the shifts in role, title, duties, and functions that the hospital/health services administrator has undergone. The hospital superintendent of 50 years ago, who was not specifically trained for his managerial role, has evolved into a university trained manager, now referred to as the Chief Executive Officer. He or she may be a member of a professional society (such as the American College of Hospital Administrators or the American Public Health Association), and may direct the total operation of the hospital.

The Commission on Education for Health Administration defines the process of health administration as follows:

> Health administration is planning, organizing, directing, controlling, coordinating, and evaluating the resources and procedures by which needs and demands for health and medical care and a healthful environment are fulfilled, by the provision of specific services to individual clients, organizations, and communities.

In the confines of an institution that definition becomes more narrowly focused. A modern hospital performs a variety of functions and activities: it serves patients, it employs the physicians who provide the medical care and staff who create the setting and enable that care to be delivered, and it provides the facilities in which the care is rendered. In the broader community in which the institution is located, the trustees assume legal responsibility for the enterprise, they provide financing mechanisms to raise funds to pay for the care, and they interact with the network of local, state, and federal agencies that have jurisdiction over a variety of activities and services.

Within this matrix, a managerial structure exists to direct, plan, organize, and coordinate all the activities. Hospitals are a labor-intensive industry with current ratio of employees per bed running at almost three to one. This figure varies with size—the larger the hospital and the wider its scope of services, the higher the ratio. The management of the personnel function alone can be a full-time undertaking.

A typical hospital has a series of departments around which patient care activities are centered. These departments may be Nursing, Pharmacy, Social Services, Dietary, Housekeeping, Laundry and Linen, Plant Maintenance, Security, Telephone, Purchasing, Storeroom, Accounting, Personnel, Public Relations, and Central Sterile Supply.

Another series of professional areas and activities such as the operating room, delivery room, emergency services, electrocardiography laboratory, and medical education involve physician services in one form or another and require interaction with the medical staff.

In addition, there is an area of involvement with the medical staff organization. The medical staff carries out clinical activities as well as education and research efforts. Included as part of this organization are the medical staff committees required to govern and to meet the standards of the Joint Commission on the Accreditation of Hospitals.

The board of trustees, as the body legally responsible for the affairs of the institution, forms another set of relationships within the hospital. The trustees select the administrator or chief executive officer who is their delegate to run the institution. A typical organization chart for a medium-sized (250-bed) hospital shown in figure 2.1 demonstrates how it is structured.

The day-to-day management of a hospital requires intervention at a series of levels. Hospital administrators typically enter the field at an assistant or department head level, move up the ladder to an associate's position, and eventually assume the position of administrator. The degree of responsibility and authority will vary at each level. A major part of the activity at all levels is to solve problems, appraise policies, and plan for the future.

An administrator will see to it that his or her areas of responsibility function effectively, that they are properly staffed, that employees are motivated, that pro-

Typical Organization Chart for Medium Size Hospital

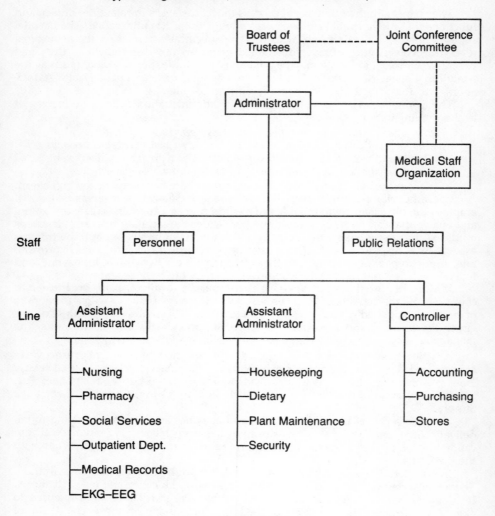

Figure 2.1
Organization Chart for a 250-Bed Hospital

ductivity is high, and that the organizational goals are fulfilled. These activities need to be conducted on a 24-hour, 365 day-a-year basis. The administrator needs to identify problems, consider various alternatives, and resolve them. Problems can include inadequate food service, complaints about nursing service, loss of medical records, lack of adequate reimbursement for emergency room services, community opposition to an expansion program, or the establishment of an affiliation with a medical school. In larger hospitals, administrators may be employed in staff roles as special assistants, coordinators, planners, community relations specialists, and troubleshooters.

Today's problems do not resemble what occurred yesterday, nor are the solutions replicable. An administrator's calendar can include appointments with the chief of engineering to solve a problem with a boiler, with the chief of surgery to discuss a professional issue, with the architect to review building design, the treasurer of the board of trustees to solve financial problems, a student seeking career counseling, the shop steward on a labor-management issue, the attorney representing the hospital in a malpractice case, and so on.

Who are the Administrators? How Did they Get There?

Administrators come into the field from a variety of backgrounds. Over the years, the administrator typically gravitated to the position from medicine or nursing. However, as institutions became more complex, formal education for hospital administration emerged and became the dominant force in the preparation of administrators for the field.

Why does anybody become interested in hospital administration as a career? Many people have friends or relatives working in the health field, while others have personal experience. Some are attracted to the field because of its increased visibility in literature, movies, and television programs relating to hospitals and health care.

The most influential person affecting a career choice is often another hospital administrator. The best way to learn about the field is to discuss it with a practicing administrator, most of whom are more than willing to share their insights.

The traditional career track, discussed in greater detail in chapter 1, is a graduate or undergraduate degree in Health Administration, a residency or entry-level job in the field, and progression through the hierarchy. Preparation for graduate training can take a variety of approaches, ranging from liberal arts to science courses. The prerequisites for graduate courses, can best be determined by a session with the high school or college guidance counselor.

The best source of information regarding the programs is the Association of University Programs in Health Administration, located in Washington, D.C. Again, I refer the reader to chapter 1 for an overview of the variety of programs.

What Are the Rewards?

As with other health professionals, hospital administrators do not generally expect great financial reward from their field. The typical administrator who spends 50 to 60 hours a week in his job would find a greater financial return for his efforts and managerial ability in the commercial world. I believe the administrator is motivated by a desire to help people and to improve society. Industrial psychologists have demonstrated that job satisfaction and a sense of personal fulfillment are essential if an establishment is to attract and retain personnel. The hospital administrator derives such satisfaction from achieving a goal, whether it be the inauguration of a new program, the construction of a new facility, or the successful resolution of a particularly difficult problem.

There are other, more tangible aspects as well. The chief executive of a hospital has high visibility, is an important member of the community, and has considerable impact in his or her executive capacity.

There are financial rewards as well. The increasing recognition of the need for highly qualified professionals has reflected itself in higher starting salaries. Chief executives are being remunerated in accordance with the size of their institutions, generally measured by the hospital's gross revenues. Compensation patterns vary by region of the country, comparative costs of living, education and background of the executives, age, and experience.

At large urban institutions with operating budgets in excess of $50,000,000, the annual salary for the chief executive might be $40,000 to $50,000 per year. Fringe benefits can include health, life, and disability insurance, four weeks' vacation, paid time off for professional conferences, a retirement program, and possibly the use of an automobile and other expense reimbursement. Salaries for associate and assistant administrators are scaled down accordingly.

19

What Does It Take to Be a Hospital Administrator?

Hospital administration is not a field for everyone. Its applicants should have certain personality traits, attitudes, and skills, similar to those possessed by people who enter the management field. The effective administrator must have the ability to solve problems, make sound judgments, accept responsibilities, make decisions in the face of uncertainty, develop and maintain effective organizational relationships, negotiate, employ sound financial management, and communicate.

The hospital administrator must be willing to work long hours as needed, demonstrate a sense of honesty and integrity in his or her dealings, be able to conceptualize and subsequently to implement these concepts, be persistent, and have the ability to persuade others to accept his or her point of view.

Dr. Malcolm MacEachern's 1935 classic text, *Hospital Organization and Management*, lists the qualifications of an administrator, most of which are relevant today:

1. Be endowed with infinite tact and diplomacy.
2. Have firmness tempered with consideration.
3. Be an organizer.
4. Be a leader in the community.
5. Have a sense of responsibility and the seriousness of his work.
6. Be absolutely honorable and just.
7. Be a judge of human nature.
8. Be industrious and interested in his work.
9. Have administrative ability.
10. Have a broad educational background.
11. Have a neat appearance.
12. Be an educator.
13. Be a good buyer.
14. Have a mechanical turn of mind.
15. Have the ability to work with others.

Today one can add to this list:

16. Understand financial management and reimbursement systems.
17. Be a planner, both short- and long-term.
18. Be a fund raiser.
19. Have an understanding of the legal aspects of medicine and health care.
20. Understand broad health care issues and the institution's role in those issues.

Hospital administration is not a field for someone without the courage to support and advance his or her principles. At times the administrator must take a position that may run counter to that of the medical staff and the board of trustees.

Sound management practices apply as firmly to the nonprofit sector as they do to business. Management affects what the hospital produces—its quality of patient care. Of course, management does not stand alone. High quality care requires the cooperation of physicians, patients, hospital staff, management, and the board of trustees. The hospital administrator is at the interface of all these elements and must skillfully blend the contributions of all the concerned parties.

What Are the Opportunities?

Today's graduates from schools of health administration are finding entry-level administrative positions in hospitals difficult to obtain. The time when virtually every graduate was snapped up by the hospital industry has now passed. Researchers have estimated that the market for hospital administrators will grow from its present capacity of 17,500 to 20,000 by 1990. This includes an estimate of a one percent growth factor, or an average yearly demand of 185 administrators to fill new positions. This does not take into consideration attrition and technological obsolescence among current administrators. These factors could account for some 500 additional positions per year.

This number falls short by some 50 percent of the current number of program graduates, and it does not take into account that more programs and more graduates are being added each year. I receive at least two or three résumés every week from job seekers.

The employment problem is compounded by the fact that current public policy favors shrinking the hospital system. The federal government has indicated that the current ratio of 4.4 beds per 100,000 Americans is too high and should be reduced to 4.0. This means the reduction of hospital size and the closing of many institutions in the near future.

Nevertheless, job opportunities for hospital/health administrators will increase despite decreasing hospital demand. The opportunities will come from other sectors of the industry, such as nursing homes, home health agencies, health planning agencies, and private industry. New types of delivery systems, such as health maintenance organizations, clinics, shared service corporations, and multi-institutional units, will require trained people. The rapid growth in the investor-owned companies that manage hospitals, the consulting firms, the accounting firms, and the auditing firms will also give rise to additional jobs.

What About Other Opportunities?

A review of where alumni of programs of health or hospital administration end up clearly reveals that many graduates make their way into related health care fields. There is a vast industry supporting hospitals and health care, made up of drug firms, hospital supply companies, consulting firms, educational firms, hospital management firms, etc. Others move into government service, health insurance companies, planning agencies, public policy roles, and long-term care.

The health field is vast, and the cross-over options are numerous. The knowledge and techniques gained through a formal course in health administration can be applied to a variety of settings. The basic problem-solving skills can be utilized in any organization.

Hospital administrators are found in numerous leadership roles, many at high levels in the federal and state government bureaucracies. Others head medical schools and health education consortia. Many are principals in consulting firms. Others run major corporations. Recent health planning legislation has created many opportunities for health care managers who lean towards regional planning.

What's the Future of Health Administration?

The past 20 years have seen a growing politicization of the health care system. With increasing governmental funding of health care, as well as the growing consumer movement, the health and hospital field has been subjected to a greater degree of public scrutiny. An endless number of books, exposés, articles, pamphlets, broadsides, etc., have excoriated physicians, administrators, and insurance companies for running a wasteful and inefficient system. A veritable blizzard of legislation has created health planning agencies, set patient care standards, regulated patient length of stay in hospitals, and reimbursement standards.

Movement to enact a national health insurance program is also evident. Coupled with that will be legislation to contain costs, allocate resources, and reduce the size and subsequently the cost of the health care system.

Administrators of the 1980s and 1990s will face different types of problems, and this could conceivably enhance their role as managers. It will certainly provide new challenges. We can anticipate the following:

1. Governmental control will increase, and opportunities for an institution to make decisions independent of the system will shrink.
2. Resources will be limited, causing a careful reordering of priorities.
3. Institutions will be grouped in consortia or multi-institutional systems to allow

21

for economies of scale, sharing of service, specialization of management, professional interaction, and cost-sharing.

4. Duplication of services will be reduced through regional assignment for health delivery.

5. Greater emphasis will be placed on effective management and the application of business techniques to solving health delivery problems. The use of computers, the application of management engineering, and the use of zero-base budgeting are examples of this approach.

The system will require highly sophisticated, trained managers at the operating, institutional, and governmental levels. We can look forward to a steadily increasing demand for qualified health administrators to fill a variety of jobs created through national health insurance.

REFERENCES

The following books were of use in the preparation of this chapter and can be of assistance as reference material for those wishing to find out more about the field of hospital/health administration. A listing of pertinent periodicals is also included.

1. Bachmeyer, Arthur C., and Hartman, Gerhard, eds. *Hospital Trends and Developments, 1940–1946.* New York: The Commonwealth Fund, 1948.

2. Brown, Ray E., ed. *Graduate Education for Hospital Administration.* Graduate Program for Hospital Administration. Chicago: University of Chicago, 1959.

3. *Education for Health Administration.* Vols. 1, 2. Report on the Commission on Education for Health Administration. Ann Arbor: Health Administration Press, 1975.

4. Hamilton, James A. *Decision-Making in Hospital Administration and Medical Care, A Case Book.* Minneapolis: University of Minnesota Press, 1960.

5. *Hospital Care in the United States.* The Commission on Hospital Care. New York: The Commonwealth Fund, 1947.

6. Letourneau, Charles U. *The Hospital Administrator.* Chicago: Starling Publications, 1969.

7. Levey, Samuel, and Loomba, N. Paul. *Health Care Administration: A Managerial Perspective.* Philadelphia: J.B. Lippincott Company, 1973.

8. Levitan, Tina. *Islands of Compassion, History of the Jewish Hospitals of New York.* New York: Twayne Publishers, Inc., 1964.

9. MacEachern, Malcolm T. *Hospital Organization and Management.* Chicago: Physicians Record Company, 1957.

10. Neuhauser, Duncan. *The Relationship between Administrative Activities in Hospital Performance.* Chicago: University of Chicago, Center for Health Administration Studies, 1971.

11. Sloan, Raymond P. *This Hospital Business of Ours.* New York: G.P. Putnam's Sons, 1952.

12. *The American Hospital System.* Papers presented at the Dedication Program of the Baptist Memorial Hospital, Memphis, Tennessee. Pensacola, Fla.: Hospital Research and Development Institute, Inc., 1968.

PERIODICALS

1. *American Journal of Public Health* (monthly). American Public Health Association, Publications Service, 1015 18th Street, N.W., Washington, D.C. 20036.

2. *Federation of American Hospitals Review* (bimonthly). Federation of American Hospitals, P.O. Box 2451, Little Rock, Arkansas 72203.

3. *Health Care Management Review* (quarterly). Aspen Systems Corporation, 20010 Century Boulevard, Germantown, Maryland 20767.

4. *Health Services Research* (quarterly). Hospital Research and Education Trust, 840 North Lake Shore Drive, Chicago, Illinois 60611.

5. *Hospital and Health Services Administration* (quarterly). American College of Hospital Administrators, 840 North Lake Shore Drive, Chicago, Illinois 60611.

6. *Hospitals, J.A.H.A.* (bimonthly). American Hospital Association, 840 North Lake Shore Drive, Chicago, Illinois 60611.

7. *Inquiry* (quarterly). Blue Cross Association, 840 North Lake Shore Drive, Chicago, Illinois 60611.

8. *Medical Care* (monthly). J. B. Lippincott Company, East Washington Square, Philadelphia, Pennsylvania 19105.

9. *Medical Care Review* (monthly except September). School of Public Health II, University of Michigan, Room 203E, 1420 Washington Heights, Ann Arbor, Michigan 48109.

10. *Modern Healthcare* (monthly). Crain Communications, Inc., 740 Rush Street, Chicago, Illinois 60611.

11. *Public Health Reports* (bimonthly). Superintendent of Documents, U.S. Government Printing Office, Washington, D.C. 20402.

3   As Mental Health Administrator

Aaron Liberman, Ph.D.

More people in the United States occupy hospital beds for mental illness than for any other category of illness. Even a limited definition of mental illness would describe the health status of a substantial number of people outside the hospital. The decline in syphilis, the increase in longevity, the alteration of hospital admission and discharge policies, the growing number of paraprofessionals, the shifts in human migration, the advent of preventive and therapeutic pharmacological agents, and the alterations in taxonomic nomenclature have all had their impact on the definition and treatment of mental illness and on the administration of mental health services.

Aaron Liberman here shares with the reader his extensive experience in mental health administration. (L.E.B.)

The expanding managerial specialty of mental health administration offers potential for professional involvement and personal growth. It offers the conscientious executive opportunities for steady advancement, job satisfaction, and contact with intelligent and dedicated professionals. The consequent psychic income is an incentive for an enduring commitment to service.

This chapter will review the characteristics of mental health administration as a specialty of health administration. Analysis of the relationship between mental health itself and the administration of services to mentally ill patients will show how the administrator can facilitate the clinical process. I will also offer comments on the academic and experiential preparation for mental health administration, and remarks on applying human relations skills. Succeeding sections will speak of the social value of mental health administration to the patient and to society at large. Other later sections will speak of the social value of mental health administration to the patient and to society at large. Other later sections will discuss ethical practices, the political process, and job mobility.

As a beginning, it is essential to acquaint the potential administrator with the evolution of mental health administration as a component of health administration. Therefore, a brief historical perspective of the mental health movement follows.

An Organized Movement

The beginnings of an organized mental health movement in the United States have been traced to Clifford Beers, who in 1908 founded the first state mental health association, the Connecticut Society for Mental Hygiene.[1] Through his personal experience as a patient, Beers had become acutely aware of the wretched conditions existing in the institutions of the day, detailed in his book, *A Mind That Found Itself*.

Aaron Liberman, Ph.D., is Associate Superintendent for Administration, St. Elizabeth's Hospital, Washington, D.C.

One of the earliest federal activities in mental health was medical inspection of immigrants arriving at our nation's eastern seaports during the period of highest influx, 1900–1920. Brand has cited the high rate of immigrant admissions to mental hospitals as evidence of the seriousness of mental illness as a national health problem.[2]

The first noninstitutional psychiatric clinic was established in 1909 at the Institute of Juvenile Research in Chicago. Within a relatively short period of time a philosophy embracing the psychiatric clinic as a social institution began to take hold. The appearance of demonstration clinics in 1922 and the founding of the American Psychiatric Association in 1927 added validity and impetus to this philosophical orientation.[3]

Mental health was relegated to a position of lesser importance in the midst of the nation's preoccupation with economic survival during the Great Depression years and later in relation to the problems of social and cultural survival during the Second World War. Nevertheless, the seeds for an organized community mental health movement had been sown.

Daniels has suggested that much of the communitywide approach to mental health began in the practice of psychiatric medicine during the war. Physicians not only provided clinical services to the individual soldier but also advised the general command about such matters as the organization of psychiatric and social services, education for soldiers, policy formation, and problems of morale. Daniels has intimated that herein was the forerunner of therapeutic communities, milieu therapy, the open hospital system, and tranquilizing drugs.[4]

At the end of World War II, the National Committee for Mental Hygiene convened in Hershey, Pennsylvania, to discuss the question of postwar psychiatric rehabilitation. In attendance were distinguished health leaders who had been summoned from throughout the nation. The committee was faced with numerous problems. Some 500,000 servicemen had been discharged from active duty during the war and subsequently classified as psychiatric casualties. An additional 1,750,000 men had been rejected by the several military service branches for failing to meet the minimum personality or mental health standards for admission. Only 4,000 psychiatrists existed at this time in the entire United States. An additional 10,000 clinicians would have been needed just to reconcile the immediate postwar needs of the country. Institutions began seriously to consider using nonmedical administrators to free physicians for more direct patient care.

Moreover, facilities were inadequate, owing to the geographic isolation of mental hospitals with advanced scientific standards, the social stigma attached to mental deficiencies and emotional disturbances, and the lack of adequate financial support. In addition, the capacity for research and training was limited.[5]

The published report of the National Committee for Mental Hygiene directed public awareness to the need for increased research, training, and services in all phases of mental health. Subsequent demands for action led to the eventual passage of the National Mental Health Act of 1946. "Under this legislation, the federal government launched a major program of support for specific projects and assistance to the States and private organizations and institutions."[6]

As a result of this legislation, the National Institute of Mental Health (NIMH), founded in 1949, was assigned responsibility for the following: 1) assisting in the development of state and community mental health services; 2) supporting research into the causes, prevention, and treatment of mental illness; and 3) supporting the training of psychiatrists, psychologists, psychiatric social workers, and psychiatric nurses.[7]

NIMH assisted the states in upgrading local mental health activities and planning programs by allocating federal funds according to population and financial need.

A Community-Based Approach to Mental Health Services

The founding of NIMH marked the official entry of the term "community" as a conceptual framework for treatment and prevention. Previously, a traditional institutional approach had been employed. Clinicians and administrators alike began to recognize the importance of fostering a comprehensive approach to providing mental health services. The change in focus added complexities to the delivery of services and directed attention to the need for competent administration and well-trained mental health administrators.

President Dwight D. Eisenhower established a Joint Commission on Mental Illness and Health in 1955. This working group assessed the nation's mental health needs and recommended a series of new approaches to bring about an improved system of health care. So extensive was the approach taken that six years were required to collect and collate the full text of the report. When published in 1961, Action for Mental Health "shocked the nation into a new awareness of the need to improve mental health services."[8]

President John F. Kennedy was deeply concerned about the Commission's findings. In his 1963 message to Congress he called for "...a new type of health facility, one which will return mental health care to the mainstream of American medicine and at the same time upgrade mental health services."[9] Congress responded to the President's plea by passing Public Law 88–164, which authorized $150 million for fiscal years 1965 through 1967 to assist in the construction of community mental health centers which were intended to form the nucleus of the new federal program.[10]

Today over 500 community-based programs funded with federal grant dollars have become major providers of health services. Notwithstanding the working affiliations that have been developed, the integration of community and institutional mental health services has met with problems and has provoked considerable controversy.

In 1972, Morgan Martin, Superintendent of Norwich Hospital in Norwich, Connecticut, cited several of what he called "big ideas" that community mental health programs had developed. They were identified as accessibility, availability, and equity of care without regard for ability to pay; provision of adequate living conditions within each program; total population coverage and an ample opportunity for community involvement in the treatment and evaluation programs; primary programs for prevention; continuity of responsibility for care; and better use of state mental hospitals.

Essentially Martin seemed to be most concerned about the overlap in responsibilities between state institutions and community programs in the absence of adequate cooperation and coordination. He also criticized the existence of state hospitals and community mental health centers as separate functioning systems. Truly coming to grips with the issues as they affected both community- and state-operated programs, he felt, would mandate cooperation between the community-based endeavors and the state hospital systems.[11]

Further complicating the matter of program development is the controversy surrounding the growth of community mental health centers. The program as originally envisaged by its congressional fathers was to place significant emphasis on prevention through consultation and education to the community of service. In practice, however, programs have usually relegated consultation and education to a minor role, instead emphasizing direct service components such as ambulatory care, partial hospitalization services, emergency treatment, and inpatient services.

Another challenge with substantial implications is the future of funding for these programs. Ginzberg believes that the country is pushing against the constraining ceiling of real resources. He suggests that because the nation no longer has an excess of workers or of capital to play with, we must acknowledge that there will not be enough monies available to practice the best type of medicine for all people in the country.[12]

Hodges and Mahoney have explored some of the problems involved in meeting the expectations of the community. They have concluded that the more limited a community's existing services, manpower, and economic potential, the more radical the realignment of these resources must be before a successful community-oriented mental health program can emerge.[13]

27

Significance of Legal Actions

Much of the current concern about quality and cost of care has resulted from several individual state and court decisions regarding the care and treatment of patients on a long-term basis in state hospitals and in other mental health facilities. In Massachusetts, for example, a 1971 law provides that an involuntary commitment to a state facility is limited to those cases in which there is a substantial likelihood of serious harm to the individual or to others. The law further ensures early discharge and follow-up services in the community.

Florida has likewise changed the thrust of its programs of caring for the mentally ill. The Baker Act, like the 1971 Massachusetts law, provides a mechanism for the return of committed state hospital patients to their local communities of service.

Possibly the most significant action, with ramifications affecting virtually all facets of cost and quality of mental health care today, is the landmark decision handed down by Alabama Federal District Judge Frank Johnson in the case of *Wyatt* v. *Stickney*. [14] Foremost in the jurist's decision was a finding that there exists a constitutional right to adequate treatment for those who are involuntarily institutionalized. In addition, Judge Johnson set forth the following guidelines involving patient rights: a humane psychological and physical environment; a qualified staff in sufficient numbers to provide treatment; and a requirement of individual treatment plans for each patient. [15]

Implicit in this historical perspective is an appeal for continuity of patient care throughout the domain of mental health services.

Relationship of Administration to the Provision of Mental Health Services

There is a consensus that more effective working relationships need to be established among the disparate programs that provide complementary and competing services to the mentally and emotionally disturbed. This is consistent with the need to eliminate costly duplication of health services. The mental health administrator needs to expand working relationships with related agencies. Thoughtful referrals, admissions, and transfer agreements between long-term care programs such as state hospitals and community-based programs can have happy effects on quality of care and on control of costs.

Implications of the Health Administrator's Involvement

It was once not uncommon for physicians to serve both as primary therapists and as administrators of mental health programs. At times they established a rigid pecking order. With the advent of the federally funded community mental health movement, the power position of the psychiatrist began to shift, and other clinical professionals emerged as clinical and administrative partners. The role of social workers, psychologists, and nurses became more prominent. Sometimes the shift helped create a breach between those clinicians who favored the traditional medical model of treatment and management, and those who favored the social process model. [16] Resulting differences of philosophy interfered with the early intervention and treatment of people in acute crisis situations.

Strain inevitably developed in many state institutions. Some who found themselves on the defensive correctly interpreted community mental health as an instrument that would close state hospitals and return mentally sick people to the community where they could live and function while receiving proper care. Indeed, this philosophy eventually became one important outcome measure of the effectiveness of the community mental center in any community.

It is desirable that the mental health administrator work with the clinical practitioner to enhance the quality of care. At best, the two should be able to give and take advice and criticism, although conflicts sometimes arise when the practitioner and administrator view their areas of responsibility as overlapping.

28

The clinician may develop a protective relationship with the patient and be simultaneously protective of professional prerogatives. The administrator may try to modify the behavior of the clinician on behalf of the patient. The clinician may judge such an attempt on the part of the administrator to be illegitimate and incursive. It is incumbent upon both the clinician and the administrator—each acting in good faith—to be sensitive to each other's professional needs. Taking precedence over all these needs, of course, are the needs of the patient whom both claim to serve. The challenge to the mental health administrator becomes one of assisting the clinician to work through clinical difficulties and circumvent organizational blocks in order to achieve the objective of the mental health agency—the best possible care for the mentally ill.

Achieving common objectives requires a thoughtful process of planning and goal development, with the participation of clinical personnel and administrative personnel at all levels of the organization. This places clinicians and administrators alike in a position of contributing to their own future as members of the agency's professional team. It further establishes a contractual form of obligation in which the planning and goal attainment process becomes an end result toward which all members of the staff have committed themselves. The services that emerge have a higher probability of representing a quality product for the benefit of the community.

Preparation of the Mental Health Administrators

The reader should refer to chapter 1, which covers the subject of formal academic preparation for all health administrators, whatever their choice of specialty. Besides this core curriculum, future mental health administrators would be well advised to take formal courses relating to psychiatry, psychology, and mental health administration. Moreover, the importance of certain strictly managerial areas of knowledge deserves reiteration here: personnel administration, policy analysis, health economics, data processing, statistics, marketing,[17] and financial management.

A frequently observed fault of the young mental health administrator is the lack of fundamental writing and verbal skills. In a field notorious for its jargon, clarity of expression is particularly essential. Excellent writing and verbal skills will complement one's ability to plan, organize, and direct a staff. This point was emphasized some years ago when several scholars representing the fields of psychiatry, psychology, and social work were victims of an instructive hoax. The speaker, a dynamic man who professed to be an expert, was an impostor with a gift for jargonese. The responses to his presentation were overwhelmingly favorable, and the resulting paper describing this folly became known as the Dr. Fox Paradigm.[18]

Other academic preparation one might undertake to secure a position in mental health administration depends upon individual circumstances and needs. Premedical students, aspiring psychologists, business administration candidates, and others who have reconsidered their academic and career goals may be found among the ranks of those destined to become future leaders in mental health administration.

The professional administrator with a master's degree will understandably doubt the abilities of anyone who has not received graduate training in health administration. On the other hand, formal education in mental health administration is no substitute for instructive experience under professional supervision in the real world of work.

Social Value of Mental Health Administration

The mental health administrator should ponder how his or her contributions to the organization reflect the stress put upon maintaining human dignity in our political system. It needs to be recalled from time to time that serving the patient is the overt, professional raison d'etre of the mental health administrator.

The social value of managerial performance is closely related to the administrator's attentiveness to details—a most important consideration as the complexities of the mental health agency increase. For example, the seemingly mundane accomplishment of cutting down the patient's waiting time by improving scheduling will contribute to more responsive and more efficiently delivered care. Better administrative practices can motivate employees to deal more humanely with patients, and can change the public's perception of today's health services as inaccessible and impersonal.

Mental illness not only affects the person suffering from the problem but also a large number of people who are either influenced by, or are directly related to, that person. Mental and emotional problems, if unchecked, can debilitate an entire family. The family can lose potential income, and their contacts with others can be severely disrupted. Transferring the disturbed person from that environment to a long-term care institution can alleviate some of the more immediate short-range problems affecting the family unit.

On the other hand, the long-term effects of losing an integral family member can harm other members of the family unit, particularly children. An agency's ability to keep a mentally ill person functioning in the community can lessen the probability of a complete breakdown within that family unit and the consequent problems with other family members which then may adversely affect other people in that community. The dedicated mental health administrator contributes to the larger social universe by establishing workable, efficient, and effective therapeutic and preventive systems in mental health.

Strengths Required of the Mental Health Administrator

In mental health administration, as in all areas of health administration, the executive needs to develop those skills that strengthen human relations within an organization. Successful mental health administration depends on the proper management of human resources—perhaps the most challenging requirement placed upon a manager. In the course of managing an organization that furnishes mental health services to its clientele, as much as 75 percent of a typical work day may be devoted to decision making directly involving employees and their interrelationships.

Invariably some employees become rankled when particular decisions affect their professional lives and their livelihood. It is prudent to anticipate people's likely reactions to a particular issue and to take action preventing breakdowns in communications. Such a management philosophy requires that the administrator solicit and include staff opinions when developing plans for a major policy shift or program recommendation. Few other areas of health administration can be more perilous to an administrator's ability to function than a failure to deal with the human needs of the organization. No academic sequence exists that will guarantee success in dealing with employees. Most human relations skills require on-the-job learning.

Every executive must live with budgetary considerations. Herzlinger has suggested that "Perhaps the most important step that administrators can take is in educating doctors and other providers of care in economics and aspects of management."[19] If providers remain ignorant about their impact on costs, they may remain convinced that only administrators affect cost of care. The potential administrator needs both to learn financial management at an academic level and to translate these academic skills into the ability to draw from his or her colleagues the desire to serve the organization's objectives.

The administrator must also assess employee performance. Rensis Likert has stated: "Clearly there is a need to help supervisors and managers to appreciate deficiencies which can and should be corrected."[20] This may be approached by developing evaluation procedures which objectify as much as possible the process of assessing employee performance. The evaluation can be used to develop a consistent system of wage and salary administration. This in turn assists the staff to view realistically their relative positions and their future with the organization.

The mental health administrator who is able to develop and implement complementary systems such as fiscal control and employee management procedures can largely chart a pattern of success for the mental health agency. This is particularly true when the financial impact of the employee's salary upon the budget of the organization is to be considered. The less subjective the management practices of an organization, the greater will be its credibility with the employees.

Another professional strength required of managers is related to ethical practices. Ethics can refer to the business, hiring, and advancement practices of the organization. Sound ethical practices carry implications that reverberate throughout the mental health agency and the health industry as a whole. Medicare and Medicaid abuses by hospitals and by clinicians have been notorious. Understandably, the regulatory bodies governing the practices of the nation's health organizations have tightened their powers of oversight and evaluation. In mental health administration, good ethics means good management.

The Politics of Mental Health Administration

The political process is nothing foreign to the world of health administration. With the advent of federal involvement in our nation's health care financing mechanisms and delivery systems, principally in the Medicare and Medicaid programs, the intensity and scope of political practices have escalated. Today health care providers engage in intensive lobbying that rivals that of almost any member of our nation's military and industrial complex.

The organized efforts of mental health supporters to influence governmental actions at the federal, state, and local levels extend back many years. But the politics of mental health goes well beyond the efforts of organized interest groups to influence favorably the actions of federal and state legislative bodies. Political activities include board and staff relations, community affairs, and interorganizational relationships.

At the board level, politics are a pervasive and integral part of managing a mental health program. In community programs where board members are selected from the citizens the administrator must respond to a diversity of views. Often individual board members represent special interest groups that in turn have several concerns in need of conscientious expression. How well the mental health administrator relates to the board of directors may inevitably determine his or her professional survival.

Sometimes training or interests may cloud the judgment of board members. In one incident a board member who was the member of an ethnic minority was interested in protecting the rights of all minority staff members. This board member was asked to serve on the personnel committee, where he could oversee on a first-hand basis all activities affecting the employee relations program. This assignment purposefully channeled the energies of the board member in a constructive direction, and in turn encouraged a responsible approach to the adjudication of most employee matters. In short, the administrator must work closely with board members in policy making to achieve the organization's aims.

Intermeshed with the board's politics are those activities which influence staff relations both directly and indirectly. In mental health, as in other facets of the health field, staff members often have their own political constituencies both within and outside the agency structure. Consequently, the rapport existing between the executive and the staff is most important in ensuring continuing forward movement for the mental health agency.

Committees are not the most efficient way to administer a mental health agency, nor do they facilitate decision making. However, they do maintain communication. Staff members who are intimately involved in helping to make the decisions affecting an organization are much more supportive of the administration.

Staff members and board members will communicate on an informal level no matter how rigid the formal communication network of the organization may be. It is prudent for the mental health administrator to recognize those relationships and to use them to further the agency's best interests. Such an effort not only maintains harmony between the board and the executive, but also produces timely and informal feedback about cogent matters.

One major problem area can, if ignored, hobble the administrator and the agency: the antipathy that can arise between the executive and the board. Sometimes when individual board members become disenchanted with the performance of their executive, rather than facing the problem on a formal level with all board members in attendance, they may choose to leak the news to the community. Such public displays can only be a detriment to the management and operation of the mental health agency.

The board's politics and community relations are closely related, since most board members belong to the community and represent at least a portion of that community. Such relationships in mental health have been further enhanced by the formation of federally mandated and state required advisory committees of citizens to provide boards of trustees with citizens' views on the development and implementation of mental health services. While this phenomenon may seem to constitute a threat to the executive's authority, if properly used, it can ensure a flow of information between the board and the community.

Another facet of community relations to be weighed by the administrator is the role played by groups such as the Mental Health Association and the Association for Retarded Citizens. These associations represent the interests of afflicted persons both before the mental health organization and its board of trustees, and among legislators at the federal and state levels.

Frequently inadequate relationships between complementary and otherwise competing mental health organizations can cause tension. State hospitals, under pressure to reduce patient census, have discharged patients before they are ready to be returned to the community. Without formal referral, admission and discharge agreements between state hospital systems and community agencies, these patients can be lost. This lack of integration is not only a source of friction but exacerbates competition for federal and state dollars. In recent years efforts to achieve better interagency coordination are slowly resulting in a more rational deployment of services. But there is a long way to go.

The new mental health administrator, then, has a chance to practice diverse management techniques which actualize the political process on behalf of patients. Included in the commitment to make the system of health care work for the people are the following elements: the positive use of board members; the mobilization of staff members to provide quality information and services; the maximization of community resources to ensure that the message of community need is present in the minds of lawmakers; and, finally, the use of interagency relationships to further the provisions of health.

Mobility and Career Advancement

In recent years mental health administrators' salaries have risen, in part due to more generous public and private funding. Occasionally the administrator may have to change jobs in order to increase his or her income. Some administrators have done well financially by remaining in place and qualifying for seniority increases. At present, opportunities in the field are numerous, with chances for advancement depending on the personal aspirations and conscientiousness of the candidate.

The modern mental health administrator must become accustomed to working and surviving in a professional care-giving world marked by technology, the political process, and sometimes abrasive interpersonal relationships within a community service structure. Armed with patience, understanding, perseverance, and optimism, the mental health administrator will successfully manage the systems of care for the mentally ill and help alleviate their psychic disabilities.

NOTES

[1] Nina Ridenour, *Mental Health in the United States: A Fifty Year History*. Cambridge: Harvard University Press, 1961. p. 1.

[2] Jeanne L. Brand, "The United States: A Historical Perspective," *Community Mental Health: An International Perspective*, Richard H. Williams and Lucy D. Ozarin, eds. San Francisco: Jossey–Bass, Inc., 1968. pp. 18–44.

[3] *A Guide to Communities in the Establishment and Operation of Psychiatric Clinics*. New York: State Department of Mental Hygiene, 1959. p. 1.

[4] Robert S. Daniels, "Community Psychiatry—A New Profession, A Developing Subspecialty or Effective Clinical Psychiatry?" *Community Mental Health Journal* 2 (Spring 1966): p. 51.

[5] "Finding a Way in Mental Hygiene," Annual Report of the National Committee for Mental Hygiene, Inc. New York: National Committee for Mental Hygiene, Inc., 1945. p. 2.

[6] *The National Mental Health Program and the States*. Washington, D.C.: U.S. Department of Health, Education and Welfare, 1965. p. 11.

[7] *Mental Illness and Its Treatment: Past and Present*. Washington, D.C.: U.S. Department of Health, Education and Welfare, 1965. p. 11.

[8] *Mental Illness and Its Treatment: Past and Present* (see note 7). p. 11.

[9] *Planning, Programming, and Design for the Community Mental Health Center*. A project sponsored by the NIMH. Bethesda, Maryland: U.S. Public Health Service, 1965. p. 9.

[10] *Community Mental Health Advances*. Bethesda, Maryland: U.S. Department of Health, Education and Welfare, 1964. p. 1.

[11] Morgan Martin, "Community Mental Health Centers: Coming to Grips with Big Ideas." *American Journal of Psychiatry* 129 (August 1972): p. 126.

[12] Eli Ginzberg, "Hospital Costs—Sense and Nonsense." *Rhode Island Medical Journal* 54 (August 1971): pp. 411–412.

[13] Allen Hodges and Stanley C. Mahoney, "Expectations for the Comprehensive Mental Health Center: The Community." *Community Mental Health Journal* 6 (April 1970): p. 75.

[14] *Wyatt* v. *Stickney*, 325 F.Supp. 781 (D.C. Ala. 1971).

[15] Robert Johnson and Margaret Fraser, "Right to Treatment." *Mental Hygiene* 56 (Summer 1972): pp. 13–16.

[16] George Meyer, M.D. Personal communication, University of Texas Health Science Center at San Antonio, Texas, 1978.

[17] Roberta N. Clarke, "Marketing Health Care: Problems in Implementation." *Health Care Management Review* 3 (Winter 1978): p. 21.

[18] D. H. Naftulin, J. E. Ware, Jr., and F. A. Donelly, "The Dr. Fox Lecture: A Paradigm of Educational Seduction." *Journal of Medical Education* 68 (July 1973): pp. 630–635.

[19] Regina Herzlinger, "Can We Control Health Care Costs?" *Harvard Business Review* 56 (March–April 1978): p. 108.

[20] Rensis Likert, "Motivational Approach to Management Development," *Guideposts to Executive Growth*. Cambridge: Harvard University Press, 1965. p. 25.

4   As Health Planner

Steven Sieverts, M.S.

Historically, when resources in the United States seemed as infinite as the nation's social objectives themselves, health professionals took pride in observing that spontaneity rather than detailed planning dominated the organizing of health services. That and similar delusions are disappearing with the belated recognition that we must intelligently shrink our hypertrophied health system. With this recognition, the health planner is coming into his or her own.

Steven Sievert's article is devoted to health planning as a vocation. This chapter distills his views on what each kind of health planner does and on how the student can prepare effectively to take on the planner's responsibilities in one of several professional settings. (L.E.B.)

Introduction

This chapter is about the corner of the health care administration field that is known as health planning—a term that needs some clarification.

Health planning, clarified or not, seems to have a special attractiveness to young people drawn to careers in health care administration in recent years. Not only have special graduate programs in health planning had little trouble filling their class rosters with able students (at least until the federal government withdrew both its enthusiasm and its dollars from the subsidy of such programs), but, to a remarkable extent, health planning has also become a career goal for many students enrolled in the more stable health care administration graduate programs. Health planning seems to have replaced institutional management as the kind of work to which many talented students aspire.

Most health planning deals with the development of health care services and facilities, much more than with health as such. It is concerned primarily with the institutional aspects of medical care: its financing, its regulation, its facility development and management, and the organization of services.

The health planner, as a citizen and as a professional, may be and should be deeply concerned about how to make people healthier and how to keep them healthy. It is highly likely, however, that he or she will make a living working at planning that has little to do with the factors that actually determine the health condition of a community: people's ways of life, occupational and environmental hazards, and so on. Rather, the health planner is ordinarily charged with adding a planning component to whatever his or her employer does, which usually has little relation to matters such as nutritional habits, automobile exhaust emission levels or sex education.

This is not to say, as some current critics do, that most medical care either has little to do with health or actively harms people.[1] It is desirable for people who seek medical attention to be well served, even while some of us are trying to change popular

Steven Sieverts, M.S., is Vice-President of Institutional Affairs and Health Care Cost Containment with Blue Cross and Blue Shield of Greater New York.

attitudes by promoting healthier life styles, more extensive preventive care, and prudence in the utilization of health care services in general.[3] It is legitimate to believe, and this author is convinced, that despite its occasional scientific and ethical flaws and its defiance of traditional economics, health care meets some very basic human needs, meets them appropriately, and provides gratifying opportunities to serve one's fellow human beings.[4]

Where do health planners work? We shall get to that in some detail later. Now it will suffice to note briefly that they tend to work in three kinds of agencies or institutions: areawide health planning agencies, regulatory and quasiregulatory agencies, and hospitals and other health care provider organizations.

Areawide health planning agencies currently encompass not only the 200-odd Health Systems Agencies (HSAs) that were founded in 1976 and 1977, but also a variety of local health and welfare councils, consortia of hospitals, and special purpose ventures such as emergency medical service councils, children's health services councils, family planning councils, and the like.[2] So long as health care demands call upon resources greater than the resources of any single institution, at the least, a latent need exists for areawide health planning by groups formed for the purpose.

The regulatory and quasiregulatory agencies employing health planners range from the obvious (such as state health departments) to the kind whose regulatory functions may not be so immediately clear, such as financing agencies (for example, Blue Cross plans and Medicaid programs) and accrediting agencies. The actions of such agencies, like those of the more frankly regulatory organizations, have the intent and effect of shaping and reshaping the health care delivery system in specified directions.

Probably the largest number of health planners work for hospitals and, to a lesser extent, for public health departments and other health care providers, concentrating on the planning of their service programs and facilities. The majority of these men and women are employed directly by such entities; additional large numbers work for the consulting firms and the architects that hire out to hospitals and to other institutions that provide health services. This preponderance should not cause surprise. There are over 30 hospitals alone for each Health Systems Agency, and about as many state health departments, Blue Cross plans, and Medicaid programs combined as there are HSAs. Hospitals, public health departments, clinics, long-term care institutions, rehabilitation centers, regional blood banks, and so forth—numbering in the tens of thousands in this nation—provide actual health services to people, with real facilities and real personnel engaged in real programs. It is to be expected that most of the work of planning gets done at these institutions, because that is the level at which decisions about developing health services get made.

What Is Health Planning?

If this were a scholarly text, I would quote a dozen conflicting definitions from a dozen impressive works before getting around to giving my own definition of planning. There is no reason to take that detour here, except to note that there are two significantly different uses of the word. The first of these is a kind of adaptive semantic mutation, in which planning has come to mean a governmental activity whose purpose is to regulate the decision making of certain nongovernmental entities. The other meaning of the word applies more specifically to health planning, but I shall deal with the mutation first.

It has become common for regional planning councils to decide, with the power to enforce, that certain pieces of territory may not be used for residential construction when such construction would conflict with a policy of preserving outdoor recreation areas or when the local sewage system's capacity would be exceeded. In the health care system, this kind of planning, or regulatory decision making, is found in state health planning offices that issue certificates of need, the legal permits enabling health care provider institutions to make significant changes in programs or facilities. It is also found in some states which set hospital reimbursement rates and in some institutional licensure programs.

This is an important activity. Regulatory planning is here to stay in the health field, as it is in land use, monetary economics, natural resource conservation, public transportation, public utilities, and many other fields in which focused governmental regulation of complex nongovernmental institutions is deemed necessary.

Generically, however, planning is something quite different from regulatory action. It is the activity that leads up to decision making. As such, it must be seen as essentially a thinking process, a gathering of facts, a testing of assumptions, a forecasting of the future, and a weighing of alternatives.[5]

Planning can be informal, intuitive, and casual, or it can be structured and disciplined. When an institution—a corporation, a government bureau, or a social agency—requires a decision involving a shift in direction or an investment of resources, we expect that the decision will be made in an orderly manner. We expect the institution's officers to set careful directions, to study the environment, and to calculate the costs and benefits of alternative courses of action.

Of course, institutional heads are quite capable of intuitive, casual, and even emotional planning, making their decisions without ever thinking systematically about the long-range consequences. This is because every institution, be it a small nursing home or a giant medical center, is governed and managed by human beings, who inescapably bring to the job their own values, biases, and foibles.

Most of the time, intuitive or spontaneous planning is perfectly all right for arriving at appropriate courses of action. It is what we are most accustomed to, and it usually works fine. But when it comes to big institutional decisions, such as whether or not to expand a facility, alter a program, change a wage and salary structure, or purchase a property, the absence of a systematic and deliberate planning process usually raises serious doubts whether the action makes sense. This is particularly the case in any field in which the political, social, and economic environment is in continual flux. It is even more the case in a field like health care, in which technological development constantly outpaces the system's capacity to accommodate and adapt, and in which public expectations are volatile, deeply held, and internally contradictory.

The truism holds that planning is an integral part of the management process. But it is false to assume that institutions with intelligent, dedicated, and industrious managements all have systematic and capable planning processes. Planning is hard, time-consuming, and often exhausting work. It is, therefore, unremarkable that hard-pressed managers superbly skilled at day-to-day administration often take disastrous shortcuts to arrive at major corporate decisions.

This is a major reason why planning has become a special discipline of its own, not only in health care but also in business, government, education, and other areas of human institutional activity. When a hospital, for example, must develop a new service, replace an obsolete facility, or invest its scarce resources, its managers need to employ a careful process to clarify goals, to think about alternatives, to study the facts, and to consider the future. The decision makers, in other words, must have the backing of a skilled and careful staff so that when an action is finally selected, they can be reasonably confident that it reflects their thoughtful deliberation of sound data, relevant values, and a reasonable grasp of the future.

This is not to say that planning and decision making are the same, or that the same people in most organizations do the tasks of planning as well as the decision making. In fact, that is rarely the case, except in the sense that the decision makers (top management, governing board, or whatever) are ultimately expected to consider the products of the organization's planning process.

The people who have to make institutional decisions usually are too busy to do the actual work of planning, just as they are too busy to do the actual work of financial management, budget preparation, personnel management, or any of the other integral components of the corporate management process. People are hired to do those specialized tasks, people with special skills and aptitudes. In the health care field, the people hired to do the work of planning are called health planners.

What Do Health Planners Do?

When health planners are employed (directly or through the engagement of outside consultants) by health care provider institutions, it is usually for the purpose of staffing a process which aims at enabling the institution's governance to arrive at intelligent, reasoned decisions related to the development of services and facilities. That process, generically similar to the process employed in other kinds of organizations, generally encompasses several distinct areas of work. The following listing is in no particular order of importance:

- Organizing, maintaining, and keeping the records of meetings and conferences of the many people, internal and external, with roles to play in the institution's decision making.
- Assembling and analyzing data regarding the institution's past and present activities, including statistics related to fiscal, operational, and physical (structural) matters.
- Elucidating the attitudes and opinions of key people related to the institution, with regard to the institution's goals, objectives, and programs.
- Analyzing the local and national environment in which the institution functions. This means looking at demographic data, the political climate, relevant technological developments, and the present and future activities of related or competing organizations.
- Tracking the regulations, statutes, court decisions, accreditation standards, reimbursement policies, and other external forces that limit or create incentives for the institution.
- Assessing the resources—financial, property, and human—available to the institution.
- Assessing the market place for the institution's services: who wants and needs the institution's services, what unmet needs do they have, and what will the financing system support?
- Bringing together people with harmonious or divergent interests that bear on the institution's mission.
- Developing and continually revising, draft by draft, a written long-range or corporate plan for the institution, including clear statements of the institution's mission, its basic goals, the intermediate objectives, and the specific strategies and programs that would fulfill those objectives.
- Formulating alternative courses of action for consideration by the decision makers.
- Stimulating continual evaluation and re-evaluation by the managers of the extent to which the institution is behaving consistently with its mission, goals, and objectives.

These are the basic functions of the planner who works for a health care institution or agency. They are deliberately phrased, however, to apply just as well to the planning job at a manufacturing company, a retailing concern, a government bureau, an insurance company, or any other organized corporate entity. For a health care organization such as a voluntary hospital, a county health department, or a Blue Cross plan, one may merely insert appropriate adjectives and nouns here and there to make it clear that this planning process is aimed at neither higher profits nor selling more shoes nor making better bricks nor arresting more speeders; it is aimed at fulfilling special health-related social goals.

What about the work of health planners in organizations other than institutions that provide, manage, or finance health care? What, for example, does the staff of a

Health Systems Agency do? An HSA is an areawide health planning agency; obviously the people who work for health planning agencies are health planners too.

This is not the place to debate the appropriateness of HSAs' roles. I have written on that subject.[6] Anybody who wishes more authoritative information may look up the text of Section 1513 of P.L. 93–641, as amended by P.L. 96–79, which spells out most of what the members of Congress had in mind.

The key factor clearly is that the bulk—or all—of the HSA's activities are advisory, not executive or adjudicatory. The HSA provides no health care. It finances no health care. It enforces no health care standards. By and large, it provides no material resources. But it does *plan*, with very much the same ingredients described previously, in order to influence the decisions of the entities that do provide and finance health care, that do set and enforce standards, that do provide resources.

I said earlier that planning is an integral part of any organization's management processes. In the case of the HSA, planning is something a little different from (but neither inconsistent with nor antithetical to) institutional or corporate planning. Where the purpose of an institution's corporate planning process is to guide and assist that institution's own corporate decision making, the purpose of an HSA's areawide planning process is to act as an external force on other organization's planning and development. The HSA's role is to influence and alter the decision making of the entities in a region that provide health care, that finance and regulate it, and that furnish it with facilities and manpower.

In practice, the HSAs' planning takes three main forms:

- *Positive or advocacy planning*, in which the agency publishes analytic and hortatory documents (called plans, with various prefixes) which urge that the local health system be developed and limited in certain specific ways;
- *Reactive or evaluatory planning*, in which the agency responds to developmental proposals from the local health system, offering advice to various regulatory, financing, funding, and provider agencies, as to the merits of such proposals; and
- *Interventionary or supportive planning*, in which the agency provides concrete assistance—in the form of technical assistance, data, policy guidance, or conflict resolution—to local entities that are facing impending institutional decisions about their future programs and facilities.

If these three forms of planning are indeed the principal methods of Health Systems Agencies (as they were of the HSAs' lineal ancestors under areawide Comprehensive Health Planning from 1967 through 1975 and under Areawide Health Facility Planning prior to 1970), then the work of the men and women who work for HSAs—*ipso facto* health planners—must be to provide their staffing.

The point is not subtle. The HSA's recommendations originate from its board of directors, the consumers and providers who represent the various community interests that were brought together to form the agency, not from its staff. The staff exists to serve (in part, to be sure, by providing responsive guidance and even leadership to) its board of directors and its councils and committees in carrying out the HSA's functions. In any kind of long run, the HSA staffer who forgets this becomes an unemployed health planner—and the HSA, while perhaps cleverly managed, will carry little weight with the institutions and agencies it is supposed to influence.

The job of the health planner who works for a Health Systems Agency, then, is to perform his or her own task, which contributes to serving the HSA's board. If one goes back to the activities comprising the work of health planners employed by health care organizations, one can readily see that each has its direct and obvious counterpart in the work of health planners employed by HSAs. We shall not take the time and space here to re-edit them to fit areawide health planning more neatly.

The difference is in focus and viewpoint, but not in kind. In fact, health planners tend to move rather comfortably from jobs in areawide health planning to planning jobs for health care institutions (and consulting firms that are engaged for help in planning by governmental agencies and health care institutions), not because they change their philosophies, but because the several jobs are much alike. In the one instance, the planners' assignments are directed at helping and supporting a board in its role of influencing the development of health care regulatory, financing, funding, and providing entities. In other instances, the planners' assignments are integral parts of the management and governance of one of those entities.

But the tasks themselves are generally much the same, even though they differ in some operational details and in the kinds of immediate expectations the planners' bosses tend to have. For example, the business of interfacing with various groups in the community looms larger in the life of an HSA planner than in that of his or her counterpart at a Health Maintenance Organization (HMO) or a hospital. If you dislike long evenings spent meeting with local citizens who have strong feelings about health related matters, you had better not work for an HSA. Conversely, if you dislike meeting with doctors and managers to help them formulate their program objectives, or if you are not interested in working with architects, you had better not be a planner for a hospital or an ambulatory care center. The health planner who works for an institution inevitably gets involved in the details of planning specific services and facilities.

If you get satisfaction out of finding and analyzing complex sets of data and clinical studies in order to gain insight into the (often obscure) long-range relationships between health care and people's health status, there probably are not many hospitals or medical centers or HSAs where you will be hired to do that for them. Your best home might be at a university or a think tank.

The non-HSA areawide health planning agencies, such as the burgeoning regional health and welfare councils, emergency services councils, regional blood programs, renal disease networks, multihospital systems, and the like, tend to have job assignments for health planners that are essentially like those of the HSAs, but more specialized and, usually, more narrowly focused. The exception to this generalization occurs when the areawide agency itself becomes a provider of services or resources. For example, some family planning councils not only do areawide planning but also run clinics and direct educational programs. Some institutional consortia not only provide planning support to their constituents but also manage shared services such as graduate medical education, joint laundries, or group purchasing. Some health and welfare councils not only suggest priorities for local service agencies but also make the allocations for regional united giving campaigns.

Whether or not a particular regional agency has purposes in addition to areawide health planning, its areawide health planning functions are not unlike those of an HSA. The differences are not in kind, but in focus and emphasis. If one takes a job as a health planner for an emergency medical services (EMS) council, for example, the employer's expectations are going to be fixed on EMS planning, with improved EMS as the indisputable goal. The planner's assignments are circumscribed by those expectations: the data gathered, the forecasts prepared, the meetings assembled all had better zero in on the EMS problem quite specifically, in a depth that is ordinarily impossible to achieve in an HSA, with its much broader assignment.[3]

The Job of the Health Planner as Regulator

As might be surmised, the job of the health planner in most regulatory or quasi-regulatory agencies greatly differs from the planner's job in a health care provider institution or an areawide health planning agency. To be sure, the technical tasks—the data gathering, the environmental assessments, and so on—are similar, but the purposes are distinctly different: here, uniquely, the planner or planning agency is often also the decision maker. The planners themselves are expected to issue or deny certificates of need, to promulgate detailed regulations, or to set reimbursement rates, for example.

Therefore, it is inevitable that the regulatory health planner does different things and is under considerably different pressures and incentives from those that are faced by his or her putative counterpart at a hospital or an HSA. The regulatory health planner is accountable and distinctly responsive to a variety of forces for his or her decisions, the most important of which includes the political structure which established the regulatory program and which usually has the ultimate power, formal or informal, to get its way.

This author in no way regrets this fact of most regulatory planners' way of life. The alternative to a regulatory process pragmatically sensitive to the demands of elected officials and other powerful political forces is often one which is correspondingly insensitive and aloof from the real world, one in which the regulatory planners' own technical skills and personal values achieve the force of law, or its reviewable equivalent, principally in terms of whether its initiation followed appropriate procedures. Technocracy may give the illusion of competence and stability, but in American society, it usually does not last very long.[7]

In the more common semitechnocratic, semipoliticized middle ground, regulatory planning, whether or not in a governmental agency, functions in a political environment. Contending groups bring conflicting pressures for or against decisions in which they have interests. Whether the staff planners are relatively well insulated from these pressures (which may lead to their being isolated from the field in which they work and from the real issues) or are frankly creatures of the political process, they differ from their namesakes in areawide planning or in health care provider institutions mainly in having the responsibility themselves to make executive or adjudicatory decisions about other organizations' plans, rather than just making recommendations to a boss or a board. This changes fundamentally the nature of their jobs.

Some regulatory planning agencies, of course, are hybrids, in which the staff planners present analyses and findings to, and administer the hearings and meetings of, an elected or appointed governmental board or the board of a prepayment plan or accrediting commission. The official regulatory power will be lodged in a hospital rate setting commission, a certificate-of-need council a Blue Cross plan board, or even a single public official, such as a public health commissioner or an insurance commissioner. Here the work of the staff planners is more nearly like that of nonregulatory health planners, as described earlier: recommendatory to the official decision makers.

The Future of Health Planning

It appears that there will be jobs for health planners far into the future. As the environment for hospitals, public health departments, and other health care provider institutions becomes ever more complex—as it surely will in this world of constricting resources and rising expectations—old-fashioned intuitive corporate decision making will become the ticket to institutional oblivion. The hospital that does not have competent planners will not only fail to adapt its facilities and programs to evolving community demands and the march of medical progress but also will stumble repeatedly in its perpetual dance with the regulatory forces—governmental and nongovernmental—that set the limits on its revenues, its programmatic behavior, and the quality and safety of its interactions with patients.

In time, it seems likely that all medium- and large-sized hospitals and other sizeable health care facilities will have corporate planning departments, much as they now have personnel departments and purchasing departments. In the early 1980s, probably only several hundred hospitals in the nation have directors of planning, although this number is apparently growing rapidly. Very few state and local health departments have similar positions; when health planners work for public agencies, few are being assigned primary functions related to the agencies' own future health programs. Almost no specialty or long-term care facilities have planners yet. But this will change, as the decision makers in those institutions and agencies come to realize

41

that without skilled help, they cannot make rational plans for their own agencies' short- and long-range future.

Some institutions—especially the smaller ones—will always turn to consulting firms for help. With federal law now requiring each hospital, in effect, to have a written long-range plan, health planning at the hospital level has become a growth industry. Some state governments, such as New Jersey, have a similar requirement; the Joint Commission on the Accreditation of Hospital Planning requirements are getting more rigorous as well. While no one seems to keep statistics on where the new graduates of health care administration training programs go for their first postgraduate employment, anecdotal evidence from several programs suggests that consulting firms—large and small—hire as many as a quarter or more of each class.

Health care executives are divided as to the net value of planning services purchased from consultants, especially with respect to the perceived results of the too common one-shot contracts in which the consultants come in to gather some data, conduct some interviews, and deliver a handsomely printed and bound "plan" (which usually goes directly into the institution's archives). This is not the place to evaluate the dubious worth of the planning services that are furnished by many consulting firms, or to make the case that the better consultants provide invaluable help to their clients. Suffice it to say here that substantial opportunities for employment for new health planners are afforded by these organizations, and that the practical experience which the many ethical and competent firms can give to young people can be useful indeed in their career development.

The current surge in state regulatory activities related to the development of health facilities and services is also sure to persist for years to come with expanding job opportunities. In addition, the federal government continually hires health planners, particularly at the entry level, but not usually to provide planning services for the Department of Health and Human Services' own programs. DHHS, like many state health departments, tends to view health planning as something which it encourages elsewhere in the health system. Government also tends to define health planning as something it does to change what is out there, rather than as an integral part of its own management and direction. Nevertheless, whether they are to support a state regulatory program, a federal/state grant program or national health insurance, there will surely continue to be many health planning employment opportunities in federal and state governments in the indefinite future.

Will health planning jobs in state and federal agencies be stable and substantive? That is hard to say at this writing. In recent years, the pattern in most of these jobs seems to be rapid turnover, both at top levels and among the staff planners. This may be unavoidable during a period in which contending constituencies are rapidly changing their expectations. Whether it is avoidable or not, it is plain to see that this year's staff in many of these agencies was not last year's staff. To be sure, this may mean that the agencies in question are hiring continually to fill positions on those staffs, which is good from the standpoint of the health planner looking for work, but it may portend frustration and futility for the people who have the jobs. Their agency may have to undergo periodic sharp shifts in direction, or they may be left high and dry when the money flow suddenly stops.

What Does It Take to Be a Health Planner?

There is surely no consensus on what are the most appropriate background and training for a health planner. The field has grown too rapidly and has attracted able (and some not so able) people from too many backgrounds to permit a uniform answer to the question of what it takes to be a useful and productive health planner.

In this author's experience, however, four basic abilities and qualities seem to characterize successful health planners. These are, in roughly descending order:

1. *Skills in, respect for, and faith in the process of planning.* The key word is process: the best health planners are adept at (and they get satisfaction out of) getting the

people who are involved in decision making to take all the steps that good planning requires. What this is, first and foremost, is a zestful capacity to organize both the contents and the human events of the planning process. What it also means is a willingness to subordinate one's own views on what a particular decision should be, substituting instead a genuine confidence in the outcomes of a competent planning process. The planning director of one New York hospital tells the true story of displaying for his medical staff, administrator, and board, all of the facts and arguments both for and against the discontinuance of the institution's obstetrical service, a decision which he initially favored. By the time he finished this task, he found himself personally convinced by the powerful logic supporting each of side of the case. He chose not to close the service, but he would have had equal respect for the opposite decision. He took justifiable pride in having staffed a process that enabled the institution to make an appropriate decision in full recognition of its pros and cons. This is not to say that the good planner always defers on matters of policy and priorities. Rather, it means that the planner's preferences for particular outcomes are less important than the skills brought to bear on the assignment at hand, including most importantly his or her capacity to concentrate on the *process* of planning: the fact-gathering, the analysis, the displaying of alternatives, the written corporate plans, and so on.

2. *A strong understanding of the realities of management.* In other than the technical areas of the job, every effective planner must be well grounded in the real world in which the institutional manager functions. It is hardly surprising that the experience gained in the classroom, in consultants' offices, in the government planning bureau, in the Health Systems Agency, is often mainly theoretical, technical, and idealistic. There seems to be no substitute for the firing line, except for the rare individual who can indeed learn how it really is without experiencing it. It is not unimportant for the planner to be skilled in the technology of planning. Unless this observer's perceptions are hopelessly obscured by his own history, however, it seems even more important for planners—if they are to play a useful role for an organization—to have a solid grasp of what it takes to put together and manage a relevant institution in the real environment. Plenty of health planners, for example, simply do not understand what makes a hospital tick: the dynamics of the medical staff, the professionalism of the nursing staff, the intricacies of the financing, the board's dedication to its own formulation of the community interest, and so on. In short, the person who aspires to be a planner is well advised to spend some years as a manager in the same field, or run the risk of being dismissed (either literally or figuratively) by his or her superiors, for the ultimate infraction: uselessness.

3. *A solid acquaintance with and appreciation of the clinical side of medical care.* What do doctors do? What do nurses do? What is it like to be sick? How are illnesses diagnosed? How are choices among clinical alternatives made? What happens in an operating room, a rehabilitation unit, or a clinical laboratory? What is a CAT scan? What is defibrillation? What goes on in primary care? What happens to patients in psychiatric units? What do hematologists do? What is in a medical record? How do doctors set fees? How do group practices function? What does Medicare cover? Many so-called health planners are unable to give intelligent answers to these and similar questions—and there is no faster way to lose credibility than to demonstrate ignorance of the fundamentals. The business of the health planner is the planning of health services and facilities, yet many people with health planning jobs have never taken the time to learn much about the nature of health services and facilities. Health planners had better know about health and health care.

4. *A good grounding in the technology of health planning.* There is, after all, a body of basic practical know-how in this field, involving statistics, health economics, health status data, research methodology, organizational theory, plan development, and the like. Much can be learned on the job, but increasingly, the preferred path seems to be to begin with education at the postgraduate level. This is not to say that the many graduate programs which emphasize health planning are uniformly strong in the

fundamentals; a few appear to be so abstract or ideological that neither graduate nor professor seems to have any interest in simple essentials. On the whole, however, many graduate schools seem to be doing better and better at equipping men and women for entry-level professional jobs in health planning. In any event, it would hardly seem disputable that health planners, to be effective, have to know something about health planning's content and technology. The ineffectiveness of much current health planning, unfortunately, can be ascribed to the weakness of the grasp of the fundamentals on the part of too many people in the field.

It should be emphasized that it is not necessary to begin a career in health planning by working at health planning. Many health planners start in health care administration, public health, or nursing administration for example, or in architecture, urban planning, social work administration, or some other semirelated field. And many people move into (or back into) live management positions after a tour of duty in health planning. This is as it should be: the skills required for other jobs in health care management and the skills required by health planners are by no means identical, but they are similar and mutually reinforcing.

Concluding Note

I have tried to shed some light on, and perhaps demystify, health planning as an occupation, as a discipline, and as a vital component of any health care delivery system, large or small. It is a field in which many people seem to place extraordinary and perhaps unrealistic faith. It is also a field with a most important set of roles to play as health system developmental decisions get made, in provider institutions, regulatory agencies, financing agencies, and legislatures, decisions that must be based on capable planning processes if reasonable and realistic goals and objectives are to be reached.

Health planning presents interesting and challenging career opportunities, especially for men and women who have the qualities of intellect and perseverance that this demanding occupation requires.

NOTES

[1]See, for example, some sections of Walter McClure's excellent study alleging that 20 percent of the nation's hospital capacity is surplus and irrelevant to health (Walter McClure, *Reducing Excess Hospital Capacity*. Excelsior, Minnesota: Interstudy, 1976), or Ivan Illich's much more drastic observations to the effect that most medical care is injurious to health and to people's moral fiber (Ivan D. Illich, *Medical Nemesis: The Expropriation of Health*. London: Calder and Boyars, 1975).

[2]Health Systems Agencies (HSAs) were formed in regions in most states as a result of federal funding authorized by P.L. 93–641, the National Health Planning and Resources Development Act, signed by President Gerald Ford in 1975. P.L.93–641 supplanted the Comprehensive Health Planning Amendments enacted in 1966, which had replaced the federal funding of Areawide Health Facility Planning Agencies after 1962 under the Hill-Burton Act (enacted to encourage hospital construction and modernization). Prior to 1962, the federal government did not fund areawide health planning.

[3]One of the frustrations of working for an HSA must be the extraordinarily wide range of concerns which the agency is supposed to take seriously, with a staff nowhere near large enough to do more than a few tasks justice. In practice, HSAs, like their predecessors, tend to concentrate on the "hottest" fraction of their pressures. They try hard to do well in planning for general hospital inpatient facilities, obstetrical services, and a few other high priority areas; no one knows better than the HSAs' staffs that they do not have the capacity to tackle the bulk of their potential assignments.

REFERENCES

1.   McClure, Walter. *Reducing Excess Hospital Capacity.* Excelsior, Minnesota: Interstudy, 1976.

2.   Illich, Ivan D. *Medical Nemesis: The Expropriation of Health.* London: Calder and Boyars, 1975.

3.   Breslow, Lester, and Anne R. Somers. "The Lifetime Health Monitoring Program: A Practical Approach to Preventive Medicine." *New England Journal of Medicine* 296 (March 17, 1977): 601–8.

4.   Fuchs, Victor R. *Who Shall Live? Health, Economics and Social Choice.* New York: Basic Books, 1975.

5.   Sigmond, Robert. "Health Planning." *Milbank Memorial Fund Quarterly* (January 1968, Part 2): 91–117.

6.   Sieverts, Steven. *Health Planning Issues and Public Law 93–641.* Chicago: American Hospital Association, 1977.

7.   Havighurst, Clark C., ed. *Regulating Health Facilities Construction.* (Proceedings of Conference on Health Planning, Certificate of Need, and Market Entry, Washington, D.C., 1972.) Washington, D.C.: American Enterprise Institute for Public Policy Research, 1974.

5

As Long-Term Care Administrator

Sam Ruth, M.B.A.

The devotion to health and youth that so typifies American culture traditionally has accompanied a neglect and even an avoidance of long-term care and long-term care administration. Cure rather than care continues to fascinate health professionals. Having grown used to the patient's prompt biological responsiveness to therapeutic intervention with chemical or surgical specifics, practitioners become impatient and eventually disinterested when pathophysiologic conditions linger, as in the elderly or the chronically ill. The practitioners' negative attitude has often been adopted by the administrators of long-term care as well. And the periodic noisome scandals wracking the nursing home industry have increased this attitudinal burden. Clearly, long-term care administration desperately needs to be competently and sensitively professionalized.

Sam Ruth has devoted his career to long-term care administration. That the field has its own peculiar attraction and potential for positive things to be done for hitherto neglected patients is evident in this chapter. (L.E.B.)

The administration of long-term care institutions is a specialty that requires both academic and experiential training. My purpose here is to portray the field itself and to discuss career opportunities for those interested in preparing for administrative positions in it. While general health care services and long-term care services draw upon similar skills, the uniqueness of long-term care qualifies it as a specialty.

What Is Long-Term Care?

Long-term care is comprised of the medical, nursing, and supporting services rendered to individuals who, because of their physical or mental infirmities, must be institutionalized for a long time—for months, years, or the rest of their lives. Chronic care hospitals, homes for the aged, nursing homes, rehabilitation units, and, in a limited way, even acute care hospitals, all deliver long-term care. In some instances, long-term care patients are treated at home.

The substantial differences existing between long-term care institutions and general hospitals arise from the differences in their respective patients' problems. A long-term care institution must consequently develop goals, an environment, and programs that can meet the special needs of its patient population.

Choosing a Career

How and when does a person choose any career? That is a hard question, and there is no simple answer. Reportedly, some parents mandate their child's career even

Sam Ruth, M.B.A., is President of the Baycrest Foundation and Executive Consultant to Baycrest Centre for Geriatric Care. He is also Assistant Professor, Faculty of Medicine, University of Toronto.

before the child is conceived. Some offspring joyfully accept the parental mandate; others, not so joyfully. In any case, if you have been blessed with such foresighted parents, then you need not read on.

Most of us, however, must choose our own careers. Some do so as high school students, others as undergraduates, and still others while working. I chose mine after finishing my undergraduate studies.

A recent survey shows that a large number of administrators, especially those in long-term care, came to their positions by chance rather than by choice: they had not planned to enter the field, they had not studied for it, but, by some twist of fate, they found themselves in long-term care administration.

Before choosing any career, you must assess your personality, your aptitudes, and your interests; then you should match these to the demands of a variety of professions. After reading this chapter you may be able to decide whether a life in the long-term health care field is what you want.

After having spent some 29 years in the field of health administration, the last 22 of which have been devoted to long-term care, I can still vividly recall my own search for a career and how I eventually found one. I shall recount for you the academic and work experiences that led to my selection of long-term care administration as a lifelong profession. I do so because my own career coincides so closely with the development of special administrative skills for long-term care. Later, I shall discuss the field generally.

After having spent four years as an officer in the United States Army, and having earned an undergraduate degree in marketing, I found myself, at the age of 27, working in sales. I was unhappy. I was not at all sure what I wanted, but I was attracted to what I, at that time, called human services. I consulted career literature, but as it happened, it was my brother who told me about the The University of Chicago's course in hospital administration. I called the American College of Hospital Administrators and set up an appointment with its Executive Director. After we discussed hospital administration and its career opportunities, he sent me to see Dr. A. C. Bachmeyer, director of the course in hospital administration at The University of Chicago, on the supposition that a graduate degree in health administration would greatly enhance my chances for success in either hospital or health administration.

Dr. Bachmeyer suggested that I postpone applying for admission to The University of Chicago's hospital administration course for the current year, advising that I first find a hospital job and learn how hospitals are run. Then I could decide whether or not I was suited to a career in hospital administration. I agreed. I soon found a job as information clerk at a large general hospital, the Michael Reese Hospital in Chicago. Within a few months I became the admitting officer. There I spent much time meeting with nurses, interns, and other staff members in order to gain a better understanding of them and of their work. This opportunity to study the entire spectrum of hospital operations proved to be an excellent investment of my time.

With my work experience and a good recommendation from the Executive Director of the Michael Reese Hospital, I was accepted for graduate work in Dr. Bachmeyer's course. Following my studies, I spent two years at the Beth Israel Hospital in Boston as an administrative resident. The residency was for only one year, but I used an additional year to broaden my experience. Total pay for the two years: $1,500.00, plus room and board. Relatively little money, but a profitable investment of time and energy.

During my residency at the Beth Israel Hospital, I heard about the development of a Home Care Program and also of a Division of Social Medicine at the Montefiore Hospital located in the Bronx, New York. I quickly arranged to spend two months of my residency program at that hospital. At Montefiore I discovered a new, humane, and economical form of health care, in which the hospital was extending its medical, nursing, social, and therapeutic services into the patients' own home: an impressive innovation.

48

My affiliation with the Beth Israel and Montefiore hospitals enabled me to study humanistic and altruistic approaches to medical care—approaches not duplicated, at the time, in very many hospitals. I was enormously impressed by the concept of total health care under which the individual received the highly personalized care that most general hospitals were not equipped to give.

I have recorded my early academic and professional training to demonstrate to you how one person built a solid foundation for his career. In sum, by 1956 my professional record looked like this: army, sales, hospital information clerk; admitting officer; graduate work in hospital administration; administrative residency at Beth Israel and Montefiore; and a four-year stint in teaching hospitals, all of which led to my realization that I wanted very much to develop total health care programs.

In 1957 I was invited to apply for the position of administrator of the Jewish Home for the Aged and the Baycrest Hospital (now called Baycrest Centre for Geriatric Care) in Toronto. This combined facility of 265 beds restricted its services to inpatient and resident care.

The then acting administrator had had little experience in any kind of institutional care. Consequently, the basic programs were minimal. Not a very exciting situation, except for its two redeeming features: excellent medical leadership, and a strong, interested board of directors. Most important of all to me, however, was the unique medical relationship and integration of the Jewish Home for the Aged and Baycrest Hospital with Mount Sinai Hospital, an acute treatment hospital. Mount Sinai Hospital was headed by Sidney Liswood, who had been the assistant administrator at the same Beth Israel Hospital where I had spent my administrative residency.

I felt that the combined facility of a home and a chronic care hospital—a total geriatric facility—possessed the potential to develop its own strong medical, nursing, and social service programs. I could also see possibilities for the development of a continuum of care that would encompass an integrated health program on ground somewhere between a long-term care institution and a general hospital. I was confident about the successful relationship between Baycrest and Mount Sinai largely because I knew that some members of the community served on both boards.

Here might be the career opportunity I was seeking. However, I knew very little about chronic hospitals, nursing homes, or homes for the aged. To learn more, I sought out people who were interested in and informed about long-term care. The more enlightened administrators had a social work background. In fact, most of them had taken graduate degrees in this field. From these conversations, I was able to glean information about yet another aspect of health care that could be incorporated into the administration of both long-term care treatment institutions and acute-treatment hospitals: the ability to relate to the social and living needs of people in long-term care institutions. These administrators had the interest and the experience to coordinate medical treatment with the patients' personal and social needs.

In a general hospital, diagnostic tests, treatments, and medical routines are obviously given the highest priority. Sometimes the medical and social programs clash. Picture, for example, a resident in a long-term care institution scheduled for a special medical procedure. Coincidentally, the resident's food committee is meeting, and he wants to attend so that he can tell the dietitian what he thinks of the food. He attends the food committee meeting, and is therefore late for his doctor's appointment. The doctor complains. It is up to the administrator to explain the patient's tardiness and to mollify the doctor.

Or, imagine another resident of the Home for the Aged, a legless woman, confined to a wheelchair. She has just baked some cookies, and, with a great sense of self-esteem and accomplishment, has set up a cookies sales stand. Along comes the infection control nurse, who takes one look and wonders whether the sales operation is sanitary. Sanitation loses to humane consideration. The woman sells her cookies.

After assessing both the opportunities and my position, I decided to leave the excitement of the acute treatment teaching hospital and to accept Baycrest's offer. At last, I was in long-term care. I knew that my managerial background would be helpful. Then, too, my personality and aptitudes appeared to be more strongly oriented to people than to technology and gadgetry—traits that would stand me in good stead.

My friends and peers thought I was making a serious mistake; "Sam, after studying and working for six years in university-affiliated teaching hospitals, why would you accept a job in a home for the aged and chronic care hospital—and, of all places, in Toronto?"

Remember, the year was 1956, and the field seemed a dead end. At that time, no undergraduate programs in health or long-term care administration existed. There were few, if any, courses in graduate schools of hospital administration or health care that emphasized the long-term care field as a reasonable career opportunity. Furthermore, many hospital administrators were convinced that nothing much could be done for people in chronic hospitals, homes for the aged, and nursing homes. In fact, such places were literally storehouses for the aged, or waiting rooms for death. I knew that extraordinary life-saving measures sometimes appeared to be unwarranted. But why, I asked, wasn't more attention paid to the development of programs, which at the very least could improve the *quality* of life for elderly and chronically ill people—even if such measures could not lengthen their lives?

Although many health administrators failed to share my point of view, I accepted Baycrest's offer, with the intention of developing the medical and social aspects of long-term care.

The long-term care field grows even more rapidly today and it offers much greater promise of career potential than when I entered it in 1956: the number of positions has increased and the prestige of positions is higher. Furthermore, we now enjoy the growing respect of other health care professionals and of the general public, because of our very real achievements in long-term institutions.

Growth of Long-Term Care Institutions

Besides nursing homes, chronic care hospitals, and homes for the aged, long-term care patients are also treated in mental institutions and rehabilitation hospitals. These latter institutions do not restrict their services to the elderly. They also accept younger people for long-term care. However, inasmuch as most long-term care is centered in the former institutions, and because most of the people receiving such care are elderly, I shall concentrate on these institutions, where most of the career opportunities in long-term care can be found.

On this continent, long-term care institutions did not come to specialize in operations for the care of the aged and chronically ill until the twentieth century. This was due to the relative shortness of the average life span. Only in recent generations have we seen large numbers of people reaching old age. In many cases, the feeble aged and chronically ill were cared for at home, simply because there was less private or governmental money available to pay for institutional care.

In some ancient civilizations, and in some not so ancient, the final solution to the problem of dependent elderly people was abandonment. In the years between 1900 and the World War II, churches, ethnic groups, and charitable organizations began to establish nonprofit homes for the aged. These homes developed better and more humane methods of care than had been formerly available in public institutions.

With the enactment of Social Security assistance in the United States, improved pension plans in Canada, and the rise in the overall standard of living of most people on this continent, we began to see some noticeable changes in the quality of care for the aged and chronically ill. The demand for services, however, greatly exceeded the supply. Consequently, with few exceptions, the quality and quantity of care given to patients and residents remained inadequate.

Legislation in the 1950s, 1960s and 1970s in the United States and Canada made medical care and placement in nursing homes, hospitals, and homes for the aged easier for the needy to obtain. Admission to these institutions became possible because more money was being paid to the aged and chronically ill, and because more funds were being paid directly to the institutions giving long-term care. In addition, the tremendous number of patient discharges from mental institutions, the inability of some families to meet the special needs of elderly persons in their homes, and the growing number of older people, created an unprecedented demand for long-term care services. During this time, we saw a marked increase in the number and size of long-term care institutions.

Many states required the licensing of nursing home administrators. Licensure imposed certain educational requirements, and, inasmuch as many people had entered the nursing home field academically unprepared, it highlighted the shortage of trained administrators. Qualified hospital administrators, either through ignorance or arrogance, felt that these institutions offered few or no attractive career possibilities. Most of the positions were filled by people with little experience or understanding of the kinds of services needed for the aged and chronically ill. In short, the field was wide open for qualified career seekers.

Characteristics of the Long-Term Care Administrator

The long-term care administrator should have all the characteristics of any successful hospital administrator. These include diplomatic skills, leadership abilities, and knowledge of health care, finance, and planning.

In addition, the long-term care administrator should:

1. *Know the needs of the aged and chronically ill, and know how to supply them.* Basic to any management position is a thorough knowledge of an organization's purposes, functions, and goals. A long-term care administrator must know the underlying causes and reasons that lead people to seek admission, how they are admitted, the effect of treatment programs, the adjustment of the patients to their new environment, the utilization and integration of many professional disciplines in treatment and service, and how a relative's institutionalization affects his or her family. An administrator must know what constitutes effective care, how to render it in order to set goals for the staff and to encourage them to set even higher goals for themselves. In short, before you pursue your profession you must understand the profession.

2. *Pioneer change.* Because this is a new and growing field, there are opportunities for innovation. In long-term care, the method of delivering services is not so standardized as it is in general hospitals. It provides opportunities to chart, engineer, and expand ways of providing care to people who may be institutionalized for any length of time from one day to many years. The longest staying resident to date in our home for the aged has been here for 24 years; one patient stayed for 22 years in our chronic care hospital.

3. *Understand public relations.* The community, if kept involved and informed of the long-term care administrator's activities, is a source of board leadership and financial support. Since patterns of financial reimbursement to long-term care institutions shift and change even more than those of general hospitals, the administrator must prepare briefs to be sent to government officials.

Families must be kept aware of what is happening to their relatives and what is happening inside the institution. Families can actually help administrators improve the quality of care to a relative because of their close personal relationship to the patient.

4. *Be a leader—a skillfull integrator of people and services.* Many residents and patients require simultaneous services from a number of different professionals. For example, a person admitted for rehabilitation after having suffered a stroke, may be treated, cared for, and guided by a family doctor, a physiatrist, an intern, a social worker, a group worker, several nurses, a physiotherapist, an occupational therapist, a speech therapist, an audiologist, other medical specialists, a clergyman, and volunteers. For maximum results, staff services must be integrated. In small and medium-sized institutions, the administrator often assumes responsibility for such integration.

5. *Be a teacher and a student.* Most of the staff working in long-term care institutions

51

—especially the medical and nursing staffs—will have pointed their education and training toward acute care. For the most part, they will have worked in general hospitals where the major focus is on diagnosis and treatment. It will be necessary, therefore, to establish educational programs designed to acquaint staff members with the special health problems of the aged and chronically ill and the different modes of health care. Inasmuch as adequate income, proper diet, family relationships, population growth, and changes in health delivery systems affect the overall health care system, the administrator must keep abreast of these factors by reading relevant literature and attending refresher courses, seminars, and conferences. In our organization, all senior staff members have budgets for educational programs for themselves and their own staffs, with emphasis on strengthening weaknesses and keeping abreast of developments in their respective fields.

6. *Understand the overall concept of total care.* All too often, health care administrators are insular in their outlook, restricting their interest to what happens to patients in their own hospitals. Long-term care administrators, however—at least those in geriatric centers—must perceive the total community health care and social services picture in order to (a) help develop placement programs for potential patients, (b) create an environment in which patients can retain their independence so far as possible, (c) bring to patients the necessary health care, and (d) ensure that patients can cope satisfactorily with their everyday living problems.

An administrator must also have mastered sound management techniques and finances, be informed about the health, housing, and social needs of the elderly and chronically ill, thoroughly understand community resources, and be able to work with government.

What Does a Long-Term Care Administrator Do?

A review of my job as chief executive officer should give you an idea of the responsibilities and activities of the administrator of a long-term care institution. The job description states that the administrator

1. is accountable for innovating, organizing, developing, directing, and maintaining all services provided for residents and patients (in short, he or she develops and coordinates the organization's programs and ensures their implementation);
2. is responsible for defining the organization's goals, and assists the professional staff by integrating their efforts;
3. is responsible for developing staff potential in order to achieve the best results and utilize financial resources effectively;
4. selects, or approves the selection of, senior staff, and approves the overall personnel program;
5. reviews staff recommendations and reports; approves the expenditure of funds directed toward the implementation of plans and programs; authorizes establishment of key positions;
6. coordinates work and activities by means of staff meetings; develops effective lines of communication in order to integrate all of the various functions of the institution (in so doing, the administrator keeps abreast of developments affecting objectives and policies, and, thus, can identify problem areas requiring adjustment and further planning);
7. works closely with the board of directors by assisting in the preparation for, and by participating in, all board and committee meetings; plays a key consulting role in the make-up of the board and is responsible for involving board members in the institution's activities;
8. is deeply involved in fund raising and the financing of the entire institution;
9. is actively involved in negotiation with various levels of government in seeking financial support for the institution;

10. represents the institution at conferences, conventions, seminars, and official functions;
11. is expected to be involved in charitable and civic activities, not only for the purpose of creating and maintaining good public relations for the institution but also in order to contribute to the community itself;
12. is expected to serve on boards and committees of health service organizations whose purpose is to foster the development of long-term care or programs (an administrator must contribute his or her expertise to other health services); and
13. is encouraged to participate in professional long-term care organizations in order to help raise administrative standards throughout this field.

Unique Characteristics of Long-Term Care

Long-term care administration in many ways is distinct from the administration of an acute treatment general hospital. The long-term care institution, such as a home for the aged or a nursing home, is a group living facility that provides a continuous stream of services of which health care is only one part. For such an institution to be effective, it must function as a part of a spectrum of related services comprising housing, home care services, counseling services, day care, and day hospital facilities. It should also be integrated or coordinated with a chronic care hospital and an active treatment hospital. Moreover, such an institution must be prepared to help its residents obtain support for both their emotional and physical needs, either through its own resources, or through programs integrated with those of other organizations. The role of the administrator becomes one of integrating the services of one's own institution with those of other institutions.

The quality of care given to patients in a general hospital is basically determined by the treatment prescribed by their private physicians. In the long-term care facility, the quality of care is related to goals defined by the administrator and implemented not only by doctors, but also by nurses, recreational therapists, social services workers, dentists, physical and occupational therapists, and speech therapists, among others. The organization of services, the breadth of services to be offered, the forms that long-term institutions and services will eventually take have not yet been determined as conclusively as they have been for general hospitals. Therefore, present and future administrators and their professional colleagues will have the opportunity to be the moulders and shapers of new kinds of services which should be developed to meet the increasing needs of an increasingly numerous elderly population.

Education for Long-Term Care

Legislation in many of the states makes it appear that a baccalaureate degree will soon be required of potential licensed administrators of nursing homes. Whoever wishes to work in a large nursing home complex, a geriatric center, a rehabilitation hospital, or a health council, should complete a graduate course in hospital or health services administration, gerontology, or studies in aging. Opinions vary about what type of graduate course can best benefit someone planning a career in long-term care. It is a relatively new field for professionals, and one which is constantly improving and incorporating different models of care.

One should, therefore, build a broad background in the principles of health services administration, organizational development, and financial management. Such a background should then be supplemented by courses that will extend one's understanding of the aged and the chronically ill. After completion of general undergraduate work, one can specialize at the graduate level. Many graduate programs in health administration and health care place little or no special emphasis on long-term care administration. Their particular aim is to offer a general understanding of the health care field, combined with a management philosophy and techniques that can be applied in any health care setting. However, some graduate schools in health administration offer elective courses or special tracks in long-term care administration and related subjects. These courses include the medical aspects of long-term care, organization of services in rehabilitation therapy, biology of aging, physiology of aging, and so on.

Some universities offer graduate courses in both health administration and gerontology. A student can combine graduate work at both schools; this is an excellent way of achieving a well-rounded education in general health services administration and in the specifics of long-term care. Some universities also offer training and graduate degrees in schools of gerontology or studies in aging. Such schools strongly emphasize sociology, psychology, aspects of aging, and chronic care.

Graduate schools in health administration, on the other hand, emphasize courses in general management of health institutions and health care organizations. Successful long-term care administrators have entered the field through each of the types of graduate schools described above. Because of the heavy demand for administrators, any of these educational approaches can lead to positions in the long-term care field.

It is essential to remember that education in this field is—as it should be in all professions—a life-long pursuit. Education at the undergraduate levels is only the beginning of the educational process. To grow in the field, one must consistently keep abreast of changes in managerial skills, the manifold aspects of the aging process, and the changing trends in the care of the aged and the chronically ill.

Career Opportunities for You in Long-Term Care

At the present time, there are too few well-trained long-term care administrators to fill the positions available. Since the number of institutions has been growing rapidly and the number of elderly persons is increasing in both absolute and relative terms, it follows that the field will require more, and better trained, administrators.

Studies have shown that 27 percent of people 85 and over live in institutions. In Ontario, Canada, data from the Ministry of Health for the fiscal year ending March 31, 1977, indicated that services rendered by such medical specialists as therapeutic radiologists, physiatrists, urologists, orthopedic surgeons, and ophthalmologists to people 65 and over accounted for an average of 25 percent of their medical practice. Yet, those 65 and over represent only 8 percent of the total population.

The elderly are using medical services at a much higher rate than younger people, and their expectations of better and more comprehensive services both in long-term care institutions and in their homes are increasing. Why? Because as they become better informed about the available resources and services, they come to expect them.

An example of much growth and extension of services can be seen very clearly in my own organization, the Baycrest Centre for Geriatric Care, that started as the combined facility of a chronic care hospital and home for the aged and grew to embrace three additional components.

As one with 23 years of long-term care administrative experience, I need not speak theoretically about career possibilities in this field. When in 1956 I took over as administrator of the 175-bed hospital, I was the only staff member who had both education and training for this specialty.

Career Opportunities

The Baycrest Centre for Geriatric Care which I administer now comprises the following:

1. a long-term chronic care hospital of 154 beds;
2. a home for the aged of 375 units;
3. a residence for the well-aged of 215 suites;
4. a structured day care program, giving care to 125 to 150 people per week;
5. a drop-in cultural and recreational Day Center with some 300 members.

Baycrest's 750 full-time employees report to department heads and administrative personnel at various levels. Present administrative positions at Baycrest are as follows:

1. a Chief Executive Officer—educational background, M.B.A., Hospital Administration;
2. Administrator of the Home for the Aged—B.A. in Commerce and Master's in Social Work;
3. Assistant Administrator of the Home for the Aged—degree in Health Administration (equivalent of Master's degree);
4. Administrator of Hospital—Master's in Education and Master's in Public Health;
5. Administrator of Finance—United Kingdom equivalent of Certified Public Accountant;
6. Administrator of Resident Suite—self-educated;
7. Administrator Human Resources—B.A. and graduate work;
8. Director of Planning and Coordinating—Master's Degree in Health Administration.

The Baycrest Centre for Geriatric Care has created eight key administrative positions. Other geriatric centers on the continent have grown in a similar manner.

Studies have shown that about one-third of the patients in general hospitals are aged 65 and over. This number will increase with the graying of our population. As these hospitals initiate a total care package for their elderly patients, they will have to look to the skills developed in long-term care hospitals. We have seen some of the beginnings made through the social service, psychiatric, and rehabilitative departments of these hospitals. As progress is made, they, too, will be seeking administrative personnel with education and experience in gerontology and long-term care administration.

Most graduates enter the field by working as administrative assistants, or assistant administrators in medium- and large-sized institutions. Others find more specialized positions, in such areas as health planning, researching, and working in health councils, government health, social service departments, and ambulatory care centers for the aged and the chronically ill. In seeking work, some graduates find administrative positions in the smaller nursing homes and in homes for the aged.

Positions and Salaries

In 1978, starting salaries of $18,000 were not uncommon for those holding graduate diplomas. To those with administrative experience, some of the larger institutions were offering even higher starting salaries.

In many of the large geriatric centers and chronic care hospitals, we have seen an evolution in top administrative titles and responsibilities. The title Executive Director appears to be used most often. But Executive Vice-President or even President can also refer to the chief executive officer.

In most cases a new title means more responsibility and authority. For example, in the large centers a number of administrators report to the chief executive officer; this status not only enhances one's position but also requires more managerial know-how. The long-term care administrator may also be elected to the board of directors.

Chief executive officers who assume such responsibilities are able to command salaries well above the average. In fact, salaries ranging from $40,000 to $50,000 are not uncommon. Major geriatric centers pay even more. Furthermore, fringe benefits compare favorably with those of industry.

Summary and Conclusions

If you have assessed your personality and defined your life goals, and you find long-term care interesting, you should then do the following:

1. talk with people who are knowledgeable about long-term care;
2. read all you can find to read about the field;
3. get some work experience in a long-term care facility (Don't worry about status. Learn and build on experience.);
4. select a course that will give you a broad background in health administration; take elective courses related to long-term care;
5. base your choice of field work on future career development rather than on the size of the stipend.

In this chapter, I have tried to give you a general idea of what to expect from a career in long-term care administration. If you feel that your personality and aptitudes fit the requirements, this could be a challenging and financially rewarding profession for you.

For further information, you should get in touch with administrators in your geographic area. You can also write to the relevant organizations that are listed in the Supplement to this book.

6   As Group Practice Administrator

Austin Ross, M.H.A., F.A.C.M.G.A.

Although group practice has ceased to be the novelty it once was, the logic of its existence remains unassailable. It benefits both physicians, who save on overhead by pooling their resources, and patients for whom it provides convenient access to the many talents in the multispecialty group. Reimbursement to the groups may be on the basis of either fee-for-service or prepaid capitation. The federally endorsed version of group practice, the Health Maintenance Organization (HMO), is politically respectable today, although a few deacdes ago its organizational structure provoked the wrath of established medicine. When clinicians organize themselves into groups, they press one of their number into a part-time administrative role. It is then but a matter of time before the successfully expanding group must hire a full-time professional health administrator as manager. Group practice is a growth industry that will continue to demand qualified managers.

Austin Ross describes the physiology of group practice administration from the vantage of his own experience. (L.E.B.)

Only in recent years has the group practice administrator been identified as a distinct type of health professional, and until recently, the literature on clinic administration has been sketchy. Moreover, describing the role and function of a group practice administrator is a difficult task, because group practice constitutes a most unusual form of organizational structure. The owner (the physician) also produces the organization's primary product (physician service). The administrator thus finds himself in a peculiar management situation, since he or she is charged with administering policies approved by a board of physician-owners, who then doff their hats and submit to those policies. This can be a fascinating administrative exercise because of the physician's well-known desire to retain his or her independence.

Group practice as a mode of health care delivery is growing significantly each year. Two excellent sources of information on the history of group practice are *Group Medical Practice in the United States, 1975* by Goodman, Bennett, and Oden, and *The Organization and Development of a Medical Group Practice,* published by the Center for Research in Ambulatory Health Care Administration (CRAHCA). The serious student of group practice should become familiar with both of these texts.

Group practice is based on the simple principle of sharing resources. It is believed to be more efficient for physicians to practice medicine together, to share staff, facilities, and equipment, and to provide each other with professional backup. However, to function in a group requires a degree of sacrifice. Instead of being the sole proprietor of his practice, the group physician must share decision-making responsibilities. In smaller groups, all partners in ownership participate in decision making. As a group grows in size, decision making is usually delegated to an elected executive committee or managing committee, which functions as a board. An administrator is retained to

---

Austin Ross, M.H.A., F.A.C.M.G.A., is Administrator of The Mason Clinic in Seattle, Washington.

conduct certain business and administrative activities for the group and is responsible to the physicians in both their roles as board members and as partners or stockholders. He or she is literally the person in the middle.

As defined by the governing bodies of the American Medical Association, the American Group Practice Association, and the Medical Group Management Association, medical group practice is the provision of health care services by a group of at least three licensed physicians-practitioners who are engaged full-time in a formally organized and legally recognized entity, sharing the group's income and expenses in a systematic manner, and sharing facilities, equipment, common records, and personnel involved in both patient care and business management.

Medical groups can be single specialty (i.e., orthopedics), or multispecialty. A majority of groups are classified as multispecialty practices (58.5 percent of groups are multispeciality, 35.3 percent are single specialty, and 5.9 percent are family practice).[1]

Medical group practices can be organized as free standing or hospital-based group group practices functioning in facilities leased from a hospital. Hospital-based group practices are not necessarily controlled by the hospital; they can be independent groups located in a hospital-owned structure. This chapter describes the role of the group practice administrator of the independently structured method of practice, regardless of location.

The American Medical Association reported in 1975 that 8,483 organizations identified themselves as medical group practices. Many of these consisted of fewer than six physicians.[2]

TABLE 6.1
GROUP PRACTICE: SIZE OF GROUPS

Number of Physicians in Group	Percent of Total Groups
3	29.0
4	23.3
5	12.5
6	8.9
7	5.5
8–15	13.5
16–25	3.8
26–49	2.2
50–99	0.8
100 and over	0.4

Source: Group Medical Practice in the U.S., 1975. AMA.

The American Medical Association also estimated that in the same year 66,842 physicians practiced in groups. This constituted 23.5 percent of all physicians in nonfederal practice.

The growth of group practice results in part from the solo practitioner's realization that it is increasingly difficult to keep up with current technology, regulations, and methods of reimbursement simultaneously. Another factor helping to make group practice visible is the shift taking place within medical schools. The medical student is exposed to the concept and consequences of shared practice earlier in his or her education than were students in the recent past. He or she finds it more natural to be associated with groups when starting practice than was previously true of physicians new to practice.

The clustering of physicians in groups is viewed by many as a solution to the problem of shortages of physicians in rural or metropolitan underserved areas. The growing use of paraprofessionals, such as the nurse practitioner who practices with physicians to extend health services to more patients, further focuses attention on the advantages of functioning as a group.

While group practice is growing rapidly in this nation, we also find signs of its development elsewhere. A recent phenomenon in Germany and England, both nations with highly nationalized health systems, indicates some growth of group practice. Medical group practice, as a significant mode of practice, is much more predominant in the United States and Canada than in any other of the western industrialized nations.

Medical group practice can be organized as a corporation, partnership, association, solo proprietorship, or foundation. While there are differences in the legal structure, the basic function of the medical group is similar. An analysis of the 7,229 group practices reveals an organizational structure as follows:[3]

TABLE 6.2
ORGANIZATIONAL STRUCTURE OF GROUP PRACTICES

Organizational Structure	Percent of Groups in Each Category
Professional Corporation	61.6
Partnership	26.9
Association	6.3
Solo Proprietorship	1.5
Foundation	0.4
Other	3.3

Source: Group Medical Practice in the United States, 1975. AMA

The management role probably varies little among these five legal forms of control and ownership.

Organizational Conditions

Some organizational conditions are specific to clinic management. A description of several of these might clarify the management role. The clinic administrator as an employee must obviously be responsive to the direction of those who own the business, the physicians. A corporate executive must have a similar relation to his or her board of directors, as does the hospital executive to his or her board. The difference is that neither the corporate board member nor the hospital board director usually engages directly in producing services in the organization. The physician-owner is on the assembly line. As an executive officer in the clinic, the administrator has the challenging task of allocating personnel, equipment, and other resources in support of the individual (the physician) who not only consumes these services but also judges the administrator's capability as an executive.

Another organizational condition has to do with shared responsibility, a factor frequently seen with the clinic but less frequently in the corporate setting. For example, the nurse works closely with the physician who provides him or her with day-by-day supervision. The same nurse is also responsible to a nursing supervisor or clinic administrator, and must conform to overall policies of the institution. The nurse is responsible to both physician-owner and administrative representative, a situation which can lead to confrontation.

Specialization is another condition. In the corporate setting, the executive is responsible for the organization's overall direction and guidance, but in the clinic the administrator operates more as a business specialist. Medical decisions are made by physicians. Yet, when the clinic administrator is faced with a problem, he or she has to focus on it not only as a specialist in business affairs but also as a generalist in the context of the organizational environment.

59

Status is a fourth condition. In working with personnel problems, the administrator often faces the conflict of the prerogative of the physician versus the good of the clinic. In many cases the goals coincide, but, on occasion, the prerogative of the physician can take precedence over the larger interest of the clinic, with a compromise in results. The medical structure is usually hierarchical, with the result that the nurse tends to have more status than the receptionist, the receptionist more status than the records clerk, and so forth.

Another condition is the conflict between the need for adequate financial return and the need for quality improvement. All businesses face conflict between dollars and quality, but seldom will you find the issue quite so confused as it is in the medical setting. Viewing the group as a corporation makes quality an important consideration, but the key issue from the stockholders' point of view is the degree of financial return. The clinic administrator must balance the need to maximize financial return with the need to continually upgrade equipment and personnel, so that the quality of patient care as well as the quality of the physician's professional life may be improved.

Profile of the Clinic Administrator

Those who serve clinics in administrative roles come from varying educational and vocational backgrounds. You will find teachers, accountants, bankers, insurance brokers, and attorneys. An increasing number of administrators come from hospitals and other health care institutions. As a practical matter, groups seeking administrators today tend to look for individuals with degrees in health services or business administration, or the equivalent in experience. Obviously, some administrative orientation in the field of health care is highly desirable. The complexities of the clinic administrator's work require a reasonable degree of intelligence; the need to work through and with others requires emotional stability and maturity. The administrator must be able to express himself well both orally and in writing. He or she must relate well to the medical staff and be capable of publicly representing the clinic.

A survey of 991 clinics found their current administrators to have the following educational backgrounds:[4]

> 7.3 percent less than college
> 16.6 percent one to two years of college
> 41.7 percent three to four years of college
> 34.4 percent five or more years of college.

Of further interest is that, of 7,606 groups surveyed by the American Medical Association,[5]

> 55.7 percent of all groups have administrators
> 70.7 percent of all multispecialty groups have administrators
> 56.1 percent of all family practice groups have administrators
> 45.5 percent of all single specialty groups have administrators.

The administrative chief of a medical group practice is known by various titles. The most common title is that of clinic administrator. Other titles include business manager, executive director, administrative director, executive administrator, and clinic manager. Whoever is employed by the group must provide a sound resource for the nonmedical aspects of practice. As a business specialist in a professional setting, the administrator enters every phase of the group's operation except the actual practice of medicine.[6] Finances, purchasing, personnel, organization, record keeping, developing procedures, designing buildings, and providing public relations all come under his or her jurisdiction.

The person who administers these functions acts with a considerable degree of independence subject to policies set by an executive committee or governing body. His or her job in the broadest sense is to provide the framework from which the physician may work with professional and personal satisfaction and with maximum efficiency. The handling of financial affairs is a primary responsibility of the administrator. To carry out this responsibility competently, he or she must be able to interpret financial reports accurately, and also be capable of developing special information from basic accounting records for analysis of the group's financial operations.

He or she is administratively responsible for the receipt and disbursement of group funds, and for provision of adequate measures for their control. He or she must forecast the group's future in terms of profitability, capital expenditure needs, cash flow, tax implications, or other considerations. The assets of the group must be protected from undue risk by the development of adequate insurance programs.

Mechanical management of accounts is another major interest. The accumulation of charges and credits, the sorting and application to the proper account, and the preparation and mailing of statements involves constant monitoring. The administrator must select proper equipment for this and other business functions, and must consider the implications of purchasing of data processing systems. An integral part of patient accounting is the processing of medical insurance claims. Here again, all will look to the administrator to develop procedures to ensure that claims are properly and accurately prepared, and that adequate liaison exists between insurance personnel and the credit and bookkeeping offices. The manager recommends fee schedule changes and monitors the charging of fees to ensure consistency in application. This means that he or she must be knowledgeable of the cost of providing services and trends affecting these costs in order to recommend proper fee changes.

Another primary managerial responsibility is the supervision of nonphysician personnel. Satisfactory recruitment, interviewing, orientation, salary administration, job enrichment, record keeping, and application of laws affecting personnel are all included in the administrator's job description. (In larger groups, personnel managers would be employed to perform much of this work.) Because of the close working relationship between physicians and other team members, one of the missions of the administrator is to ensure equitable treatment of all personnel, and this can be a difficult task. It is the administrator's responsibility to consider the group as a whole and to administer the personnel policies fairly in that light.

In addition to primary areas of business, finances, patient records, and personnel, the administrator must oversee medical record procedures, timely procurement of supplies and equipment and, of course, building and facility maintenance.

Any successful medical group participates in the activities of the community in which it is located. Along with the medical staff, the administrator bears a share of responsibility with respect to civic affairs. The clinic's image in the public eye is, in many ways, the administrator's concern. He or she must be conscious of the overall appearance of the clinic and aware of the manner in which patients are received by both lay and professional personnel.

Form letters, instruction sheets, signs, and other forms of written communication with patients are subject to the administrator's review and editing as these help to create the clinic's image. The clinic administrator is unique in the field of health care administration in terms of his or her close relationship to physicians, understanding of them, and ability to bridge gaps of understanding between the profession and the lay public. The administrator should be alert for any positive opportunity to present the clinic and its staff in the most favorable light possible.

Management needs are related to an organization's size and complexity. A three-physician group has different needs than a group with a hundred physicians. In the smaller group, the administrator has to cover many bases. In the larger group, department heads accomplish certain specialized functions. Regardless of the size of the group, certain common requirements exist, most of which can fit under five categories.

1. *Technical competence.* The administrator must have a thorough knowledge of good business practices. In a smaller group he or she must be particularly astute in accounting. In a larger group the administrator need not be an accountant, but must

be very familiar with accounting matters and be capable of supervising accounting techniques. He or she must not only be a good businessperson but also technically competent in a number of subjects.

Dr. Stanley Custer, past president of the American Group Practice Association, summarized the technical competence required of the medical group administrator as follows:

> His role is very clear. He is the custodian of property and equipment. He is head accountant and bookkeeper. He is the personnel director. He is economist and financier. He is a public relations expert, architect, engineer, politician, policeman, purchasing agent, psychologist, traffic manager, efficiency expert, investment counselor, legal advisor, insurance advisor, janitor.[7]

2. *Resource management.* In addition to technical competence, the administrator must be a manager. He or she must anticipate problems, apply analytical techniques to identify potential solutions, know when and how to make a decision, and be capable of marketing a decision to obtain group endorsement or agreement. He or she must be capable of implementing change.

3. *Communications.* The administrator must have a refined ability to communicate both in writing and orally. He or she must be emotionally under control, and cannot afford the luxury of being abrasive in working with others. As a communicator, the administrator must be tuned to nonverbal signals and be sensitive to the complex relationships between team members (physicians, nurses, receptionists, and others). A highly developed writing skill is desirable because of the need to convey matters of importance to the physicians and others, and the difficulty of gathering all parties to talk. Actions taken by executive committees, advisory committees, or other groups must be conveyed accurately in writing and in readable form.

4. *Leadership.* In a group practice setting, where authority is often earned rather than inherited, the administrator must be a pacesetter and an effective leader. The group practice administrator can expect to put in long hours. The physician's long day must usually be matched by the group's administrator. Of course, leadership is an elusive quality. Recognition as a leader in a group practice setting comes slowly, after an apprenticeship period.

5. *Initiation of change.* A fifth quality is also particularly vital to the administrator of a group that is growing in size and complexity. The administrator must be an innovator if the group is successfully to modify its practices in order to meet new conditions. The administration must not only be able to meet new change demands but also convince others of the need to change.

Compensation for the Group Practice Administrator

Administrators are usually compensated with a salary or an amount based on a percentage of profits salary arrangement. In many groups, the administrator is paid a salary plus a percentage of net profit as an incentive. Salaries for administrators vary widely according to size of the group and degree of responsibility. The size of the group alone, however, is not absolutely correlated with compensation. To date, only limited studies on compensation have been conducted, and it is difficult to draw definitive conclusions. It is also difficult to compare compensation among group practice administrators, hospital administrators, and other health professionals until such time that adequate studies of responsibilities providing cross-comparisons can be made. Individuals entering group practice have indicated that compensation is competitive with entering levels in hospitals.

Key Relationships

Some special relationships exist between the clinic administrator and members of the medical staff, the governing board, employees, and colleagues. Exploring several of these relationships may be valuable because they tell us something about the subtleties of the clinic administrator's life.

1. *The administrator and the medical staff.* While the administrator does not carry medical responsibility for the functioning of physicians within the group, he or she is involved in matters which indirectly affect the quality of medicine practiced. He or she assists in the mechanics of recruiting and orienting new staff members. Employment relationships between staff members (partnership agreements, bylaws, etc.) are developed with the assistance of the clinic administrator. The administrator has a responsibility for compiling information regarding medical staff policies.

Beyond these functional relationships, the physician and the administrator form personal ties. The administrator may advise the physician in the conduct of both professional and personal business affairs. What are current interest rates for borrowing money for buying a new home? What does the practice economy look like in the year ahead? Which expenses are tax deductible? Needless to say, the astute administrator is careful about giving advice on subjects about which he or she knows little. A mature group will view the administrator as a colleague—a specialist in business, but nevertheless a full participant in the group activities.

2. *Governing boards.* One difference between clinic management and hospital management lies in the relationship of the administrator to the governing board. In the hospital setting, the chief executive officer is responsible to the governing board for all actions taking place within the hospital. The chief of staff (a physician) usually reports to the governing board indirectly through the administrator rather than directly.

In the group practice setting, the administrator is employed by the group practice governing body, but in this instance, the administrator has more limited responsibilities than his or her counterpart, the hospital administrator. He or she is responsible for administrative services provided within the group practice setting (business office, medical secretaries, records, etc.) and collaborates with physicians in accomplishing the goals of the group practice. However, unlike the hospital's executive officer, he or she does not usually carry overall responsibility for the functioning of the organization.

In group practice, the clinical chiefs of departments are responsible for the medical conduct of their own areas, and the executive committee consists of physicians, unlike a hospital's governing board, which is frequently made up of a majority of nonphysicians.

In summary, then, the role of the group practice administrator with respect to the governing body is as a specialist in administration rather than as an executive officer in charge of the overall operation. The hospital administrator's responsibilities are broader, including all of the activities that take place within the hospital structure.

3. *Colleagues and subordinates.* Relationships with colleagues and subordinates are usually determined by the management style of the executive. Generally the clinic administrator will tend to be closer to subordinates than would be the administrator of a similarly sized hospital. One theory (untested) suggests that the clinic administrator must rely more on his or her persuasive powers to accomplish results and must function in a more democratic and less structured fashion than the hospital administrator, who must establish more formal relationships with all parties, including medical staff, colleagues, and subordinates. This creates a transitional problem for hospital administrators who change to a group practice setting. Clinic administrators tend to operate more commonly on a first name basis, relying more on informal lines of communications than can their counterparts in hospitals. Yet, while clinic administrators can function with more informality, they must somehow maintain a certain distance.

Several other factors differentiate clinic and hospital administrators, and these can account for the subtleties involved in defining the clinic administrator's position. The clinic administrator on the average operates out of a smaller unit. The average number of physicians in all groups is 7.7; multispecialty groups average 13.2 physicians, single specialty groups 5.1 physicians, and family practice groups 4.4 physicians.[8] He or she is not surrounded with as much management depth as is the hospital administrator. The clinic administrator is also under more direct fire because he or she is accountable to the individual physician within the group, each of whom grades his or her performance. The typical clinic administrator is the captain of the administrative ship, but, surrounded by many admirals, it can be a lonely job.

The hospital administrator may be protected somewhat since he or she reports to a board of directors (often outsiders) who are not always well versed in internal operating problems. This administrator-board relationship can sometimes shield a hospital administrator who crosses swords with a physician.

The clinic administrator is protected, too, but in a different way. Clinic managers administer policies set by the clinic board; therefore, physicians who may be antagonistic to a new policy or procedure must look to their physician colleagues for change, not to the clinic administrator.

Another problem can occur in communities with more than one hospital. Where physician can admit his or her patients to any one of several hospitals, the hospitals' administrators will wish to compete for such patients. As a result, they will tend to keep their distance from neighboring administrators.

However, there is a general absence of competition among clinic administrators, who share considerable information with one another. This is perhaps due to the administrator's need to keep up to date, in order to ensure that physicians in his or her group are reasonably well informed. He or she is therefore encouraged to share more than his or her counterpart in the hospital.

Management Style

Basically, the administrator functions as an allocator of resources. He or she serves as a coordinator, an innovator, and a steward. This stewardship involves developing and implementing policies and procedures, and monitoring the organization. The administrator's leadership is accomplished by the consent of others. His or her authority is structural, but by nature he or she tends to surmount conflict or controversy by seeking compromises, presumably equitable ones. To be a successful leader and innovator, the administrator needs to have a base of good will and respect. The skill of leading through persuasion from a reservoir of good will and respect is perhaps a keystone of the practice of administration in groups.

Administrators operating within the group practice setting must be equipped with a high degree of interpersonal sensitivity. To create an environment in which change will be accepted by the physicians, the administrator must first move the medical leadership to endorse and support such change rather than to claim it as the prerogative of a title or position.

Does this imply that administrators must be timid? Is the decision-making process so slow that decisions must be deferred until the environment is ripe for change? In reflecting on these relationships, are you left with a vision that our group practice administrators must wear green shades and sit in their business offices safely surrounded by their ledgers?

Emphatically, no. To overcome some of these organizational obstacles requires a distinct element of courage. Fortunately, most physicians recognize instinctively the administrator's difficulty in the group practice setting, and many group administrators have attested to the fact that special bonds develop between administrators and physicians. The physician is in an excellent position to monitor the end result of the administrator's performance, and once the physician staff are comfortable with the administrator (and vice versa), a strong relationship blossoms which allows the administrator to move more easily into decision making. But if you are an ambitious administrator who needs to receive top organizational billing, you would be well advised to stay away from group practice. A physician elected as chairman of the board (or executive or managing committee) quite properly is the person at the top of the ladder.

As a business specialist, the administrator must also fulfill a role as a conservator

64

of the partnership or practice interest. It is the administrator who must often point with concern to the tendency to overexpand or to buy too much equipment or facilities. It is the administrator who must worry with the physicians about the adequacy of their medical liability insurance coverage or, for that matter, insurance to cover all of the other potential and catastrophic incidents ranging from embezzlement to disasters of a more natural variety. It is often the administrator who plays the quiet counseling role for the young physician who finds him- or herself financially overextended. In addition to the obvious accounting and business practices, the administrator, then, must also exercise a fully matured sense of discretion.

The Administrator as a Human Resource Expert

One of the administrator's greatest challenges relates to the successful application of human resources in support of the clinic's mission. The recruiting of team members to support the physician is on the list of essential functions. Group practice is inherently a combination of dozens of mini-teams, consisting of physicians and office assistants, of record personnel, of business office staff, of laboratory and radiology technologists. On the average, four or five employees will be hired for every physician in the group. The development of team work oils the machinery and supports the objectives of quality patient services. This is where the properly motivated administrator can really shine. His or her knowledge of the physician owners' personal characteristics together with sensitivity in attracting and motivating paraprofessional staff members is a key ingredient to the organization's success. Likewise, the ability to work out differences of opinion and to know when to force change is critical to the administrative processes. The group practice administrator seems always to be much closer to the employee force than one would expect in such a complex structure.

Personnel Administration

Personnel administration is obviously a critical function. The description of several almost classic problems may provide insight to the student contemplating involvement in the group practice field.[9]

1. The first of these problems is rebellion against central authority. At the very root of personnel problems affecting the professional staff, the nurses, and other employess is a very constant and subtle motion toward rebellion against central management. In few other businesses can you expect to encounter such subtle but constant warfare in which the manager gets caught in the middle.

The equitable enforcement of clinic policies and procedures in the name of the group is one of the more trying tasks of our administrator. How does the administrator cope with the physician who wants to give his or her *own* nurse a little extra time off or a little extra money, while several hundred other employees who do not have close liaison with any of the physicians are compelled to follow the standard personnel policy? One of the neophyte administrator's first lessons is learning to cope with rebellion against central management or authority.

2. A second classic conflict occurs between members of the professional staff. Here the administrator faces a particularly dangerous situation. Physician A comes to the administrator with a beef about Physician B. If the administrator identifies with Physician A, Physician A feels comfortable about the situation and tends to look with favor on our administrator. Ultimately, however, Physician B will later arrive on the scene to register some complaints or concerns about the policies or approaches of Physician A. If our administrator now identifies and sympathizes with Physician B, it will be a relatively short time before Physician A and Physician B discover that the only thing they have in common is the belief on the part of each that the administrator identifies with *his*, or *her*, side of the story. Yet the administrator, when approached by either physician, cannot simply answer "This doesn't involve me—go take your complaints elsewhere." No, the administrator has to listen and has to be skillful

enough to interpret the facts, and even offer some advice toward reconciling their differences.

Maintaining the necessary objectivity and impartiality is not easy to do, particularly when it would be easiest to agree with the physician who happens to be in the office. You have to develop some good listening postures, which cannot be learned from a book. Conflicts between members of the professional staff are very quickly picked up by other employees in the clinic, and a very important function of the clinic administrator is to minimize inevitable intra-professional conflicts.

3. A third classic problem is the employee who is seeking special status. A status seeker emerges when a highly intelligent, well-motivated employee begins to take on the physician's mantle when dealing with others. For the political animal, a clinic structure can be a fool's paradise. The higher the physician is in the professional structure, the higher the prestige of those working directly with him or her. There are some, although fortunately few, who play this game to the detriment of not only other personnel but also physicians. The highly efficient office assistant or secretary who is accidentally coupled with a physician who fails to recognize that this assistant is misusing power can create a difficult situation for our administrator. Picture if you would the clinic administrator's nightmare of a twenty man group, with each physician staffed with twenty assistants who believe that the end justifies the means in order to make her phsyician's life happier (and her own). Disruptive action taken by employees in the name of the physician cannot be ignored, but must be approached gingerly, carefully, but effectively.

4. The fourth of our classic problems occurs when the administrator attempts to adjudicate patient complaints. These situations, in which, for example, a patient complains to the administrator about a physician's or nurse's performance, require unusual tact and perception. Let us assume the long-time patient has complained that the nurse was intentionally rude. Our naive administrator may hastily assume that the patient is always right and may attempt to take direct and immediate action to inform the physician's nurse of this situation and to look for immediate improvement. But perhaps the administrator has better review the situation carefully before drawing any premature conclusions. It might well be that the patient is a chronic complainer, or it might also be that the physician was encouraging the nurse to turn the patient off. In any case, the administrator is caught in the middle and must critically balance the elements of each situation.

5. The fifth of our classic problems occurs when the administrator has to face unrealistically high expectations from members of the medical staff. To understand this particular classic, we should remind you that when the physician wishes to solve a patient problem, he or she is in a position to gather the facts (laboratory tests, x-ray, and so forth) and to act personally on those facts. The physician is close to the scene (the patient) and has considerable control over the factors which bring about the change in the patient's condition. Failure of those around him or her to respond to orders for patient treatment or care can be dealt with quickly and usually, effectively. This is as it should be. The administrator, on the other hand, in order to solve his or her problems, usually has to work *through* other people, often the physician. The administrator's role and status is earned and not inherited. This leads to a certain degree of frustration on the part of both the physician and the administrator. For example, the physician may complain because too many of the medical records arrive late for patient appointments. He or she complains to the administrator and expects instant results. The administrator, on the other hand, realizes that one of the reasons these charts are arriving late is because they are held up in another doctor's office or elsewhere in the system. To solve the problem persuasion is needed, not authority. Often too many steps exist in the procedural sequence to enable the administrator personally to solve the problem. He or she must rely on others, and the ability to motivate these others to change depnds on many variable factors. The physician, however, does not necessarily sympathize with slow response. He or she may recog-

nize that the problem is complex, but still expect that the rabbit can be pulled out of the hat in time. The physician who wants something accomplished can be unsympathetic with an organizational need to coordinate this request for service with four dozen other such requests.

The method the administrator uses to respond to this high level of expectation can create substantial personnel problems of its own. Out of sheer frustration, our administrator may attempt to be highly autocratic, which in turn can force greater confrontation between the clinic structure and the individuals within that structure.

Advantages of Being a Group Practice Administrator

In spite of the classic problems outlined above, however, this can be a rewarding profession. Perhaps its most important advantage is the satisfaction an administrator derives from using management expertise to help physicians accomplish patient-related objectives and goals. The administrator is viewed by physicians as an important member of the team. Close identity with the physicians also tends to produce a healthy level of personal compensation. Physicians generally respect the clinic administrator's expertise, and once the administrator has proven his or her worth, physicians will solicit judgment and counsel. This is a satisfying relationship.

The challenge of group practice administration lies in the need to communicate persuasively with many different people. The administrator tends to be closer to the operating problem level than is the administrator of the hospital of equivalent size, who must operate more through department heads. Thus, for an individual who likes to be close to the firing line, group practice can be highly satisfying.

Disadvantages of Administration in Group Practice

There are also some disadvantages, particularly when group practice administration is compared with hospital management. The group practice administrator's performance is subject to constant day-by-day evaluation. Sometimes this evaluation is less than rational. Each physician tends to judge the administrator's competency from personal observations. The administrator is vulnerable as a decision maker and must carefully and continually assess the impact of his or her decisions on a number of physicians. It is impossible to keep everyone happy all of the time. Group physicians operate most of their professional lives within the clinic, in contrast to other physicians, who visit their patients in the hospital but do not spend the majority of their time there. Another disadvantage is that there is very little coasting time available to the clinic administrator. He or she is subject to frequent interruptions and must respond quickly to a wide variety of requests. The clinic administrator must become much more deeply involved in details of the operation than would his hospital counterpart. This in part is caused by the scale of the clinic operation.

Finally, the clinic administrator frequently lacks the support of department heads who are trained in supervisory techniques. In the clinic setting, the department head is frequently a technical specialist first and a supervisor second.

A Word of Warning

Executive obsolescence is a particularly hazardous area for the clinic administrator. The health industry is the third largest industry in the nation. Changes which have taken place in the health field over the last ten years stagger the mind. The development of new medical technology, changes in political and social health issues, and the proliferation of federal and local regulations have already tested administrators in hospital settings. Some of these changes have affected clinic administrators, but to date they have been protected from many of them. These changes in health care will have a great impact on clinic administration in the several years ahead, and clinic administrators will need to prepare to cope with this accelerated change.

Cost containment measures affecting hospitals will soon affect the practice of medicine in clinics. Regulations will be expanded to cover acquisition of major pieces of equipment. Patterns of change in the education of health professionals will create further separation of functions between physicians and other medical team personnel. Specialization and fragmentation will create additional challenges for the clinic administrator. Patients now are exposed to dozens of technical personnel, which can change attitudes about personalization of health care. (It was not too long ago that those involved in group practice would have thought it impossible to pass a law requiring physicians to monitor other physicians on the quality of care. Few predicted the extent of the environmental and consumer movements' impact.) While the hospital administrator's life has been seriously affected for some time by the need to participate on regional health planning councils, budgeting task forces, or meetings with city planners and consumer advocates, these pressures have not yet been experienced by the clinic administrator.

The Joint Commission on Accreditation of Hospitals has made significant changes in the hospital setting, and the new ambulatory care accreditation program jointly sponsored by the Joint Commission on Accreditation of Hospitals, the American Group Practice Association, the American Medical Association, and the Medical Group Management Association, will add additional pressures (even though these are benevolent forces). The group practice administrators of the future will face these problems, along with the changing attitudes of patients, and they had better be prepared to work diligently to avoid personal obsolescence.

Summary

We find the clinic administrator quite often caught in the middle. He or she is involved in a peculiar organizational framework with special working conditions. Clinic administrators must promote the welfare of a centralized clinic operation while minimally affecting the individual liberties and prerogatives of its owners. They must deal fairly and impartially with individual employees, even though physician supervisors may not always support them wholeheartedly.

As in Merlin's Magic Shop in Disneyland, clinic administrators must have at their fingertips a wide variety of mysterious tools and techniques to assist in lubricating the decision-making machinery; but while doing so, they must be neither wily nor shrewd. They will always be expected to be honest magicians. The administrator must know how and when to compromise. And while doing all this, he or she must learn to climb out from those well shafts, sinkholes, and swamps without acknowledging having fallen in over his or her head. The clinic administrator is his or her own counselor, and if things are not going well, this can be a very lonely world indeed.

The clinic is a world that provides you with an opportunity to demonstrate your skills and to gain the satisfaction of knowing that you are working on a one-to-one basis with a group of very highly motivated and intelligent people. In spite of all of its problems, the clinic setting is one of the most invigorating and satisfying settings possible—even if the administrator seems always to be caught between competing and conflicting forces.

NOTES

[1] American Medical Association, Center for Health Services and Delivery, *Group Medical Practice in the U.S., 1975.* pp. 4, 10, 12, 13.

[2] *Ibid.,* pp. 4, 10, 12, 13.

[3] *Ibid.,* p. 49.

[4] Medical Group Management Association, Denver, Colorado, 1977.

68

[5]American Medical Association, *Group Medical Practice in the U.S., 1975.* p. 56.

[6]Fred E. Graham, Ph.D. (Associate Director, Medical Group Management Association, Denver, Colorado), "The Medical Group Manager," (unpublished).

[7]G.S. Custer, "The Role of the Administrator in Group Practice," *Medical Group Management* 19, 1 (November 1971):4-5E.

[8]American Medical Association, *Group Medical Practice in the U.S., 1975,* p. 12.

[9]Austin Ross, "The Manager in the Middle in Personnel Problems," *Medical Group Management* 23, 3 (March-April 1976).

REFERENCES

Abernathy, W.J., et al. *The Management of Health Care.* Cambridge, Massachusetts: Ballinger, 1976.

Center for Research in Ambulatory Health Care Administration. *The Organization and Development of a Medical Group Practice.* Cambridge, Massachusetts: Ballinger, 1976.

Digest of Medical Group Employment Contracts and Income Distribution Plans. Denver: Medical Group Management Association, 1974.

Hirsh, B.D. *Business Management of a Medical Practice.* St. Louis: C.V. Mosby, 1964.

International Directory of the Medical Group Management Association, 1976-1977. Denver: Medical Group Management Association, 1976.

Manning, F.F. *Medical Group Practice Management.* Cambridge, Massachusetts: Ballinger, 1977.

JOURNAL ARTICLES AND PROFESSIONAL PAPERS

Allison, R.F. "The Role of the Medical Group Manager, *Medical Group Management* 22, 2 (January–February 1975):28-29.

Barry, W.D. "What to Expect from Your Clinic Manager." *Group Practice* 15, 5 (May 1966):339-41.

Brown, J.W. "Problems of Authority in 269 Group Medical Clinics in the United States and Canada. Professional paper. Denver: American College of Medical Group Administrators, 1966.

Custer, G.S., and C.T. Hardy. "Doctor Assesses Manager, Manager Assesses Medical Director." *Group Practice* 21, 8 (December 1972):6-10.

"Encouragement for New Medical Group Manager." *Medical Group Management* 20, 2 (January–February 1973):31.

Frederickson, G.K. "Criteria for Determining When the Position of Clinic Manager Should Be Established." Master's Thesis, University of Iowa, Hospital and Health Administration Program, June 1965.

Hardy, C.T. "Administrative Management." *Medical Group Management* 23, 4 (May-June 1976):22-25.

Juhn, D.S., M.M. Leboeuf, and F.F. Manning. "Motivation and Need Satisfaction of Clinic Managers." *Medical Group Management* 21, 4 (May–June 1974):14-16.

Ross, A. "Personal Strategy for Survival." *Medical Group Management* 22, 3 (March–April 1975):24-28.

Sheldon, A. *Organizational Issues in Health Care Management.* New York: Spectrum Publications, Inc., 1975.

Starr, D. "Your Manager's Style." *Group Practice* 21, 3 (July 1972):15–17.

Full list on the clinic administrator is available from:
Library Reference Service
Medical Group Management Association
4101 East Louisiana Avenue
Denver, Colorado 80222

7   As Rural Health Administrator

David H. Jeppson, M.P.H.

Most books, monographs, and papers on health administration almost routinely orient themselves toward programs and issues associated with urbanization. The exclusiveness of this attention reflects the more than 100 years of population shift from rural to urban areas—a process fostered in part by the dynamics of industrialization and the mechanization of farm work. However, rural America still has a residual population that has resisted the blandishments of metropolitan life. Moreover, there is some evidence that the rate of rural depopulation has decreased, and that in some areas the trend may even have reversed itself. But, whether or not this constitutes a national trend, the need for efficient and effective health services in rural America is apparent. Health administrators can fill this need. Each specialty of health administration familiar in the urban environment has so far developed its generic counterpart in rural health administration. The differences that do exist reflect the imperatives of rural life.
David H. Jeppson, who has worked in rural areas, discusses these differences. (L.E.B.)

Introduction

Opportunities for trained, capable young people who are interested in careers in rural health have increased substantially, and related training requirements have broadened and intensified accordingly. Administrative posts are to be found today in the rural hospital, nursing home, medical group practice, health maintenance organization (HMO), private and public mental health institution, minimum care center for the aged, and community health center. Rural health planners are in demand as a result of Health Systems Agency legislation. In addition, there are administrative civil service positions in rural public health departments and rural extension services of medical schools, state health departments, and large urban health organizations.

Rural Hospital Administration

Just under 25 percent, or about 1,700, of the country's 7,000 acute care general hospitals are small institutions of under 50 beds, and the majority of these provide care in a variety of rural areas.[1]

The number of acute care general hospitals for the nation as a whole is expected to decline in the next two decades. Less clear is the extent to which the numbers of rural hospitals will decrease. Many rural hospitals are located in isolated and sparsely populated areas, and there is evidence that national and state governmental policy will be to keep these institutions viable in recognition of their critical role.[2] The community views a rural hospital not only as a health promoting facility but as a major employer and economic mainstay.

Rural hospital boards are generally conservative and relatively unsophisticated. As a result, they tend to constrain salary raises. But as the job of managing the rural

---

David H. Jeppson, M.P.H., is Executive Vice-President of Intermountain Health Care, Inc., in Salt Lake City, Utah.

hospital has become more complex, salary and fringe benefits have tended to improve, with rural hospital administrators receiving incomes as large as or larger than those of local educational administrators and governmental agency administrators.

Individuals with demonstrated success at the assistant and associate administrator levels in the larger hospitals have a splendid chance to advance. In the smaller hospitals, administrators may work through a job or two before transferring to a staff position in one of the larger hospitals. Job availability is usually best known by professional health recruiting and placement firms, by national, regional, and state hospital associations, by university hospital administration program personnel, by multihospital system organizations, and by the rural hospital administrators themselves.

Many small rural hospitals cannot survive financially on an independent basis because their patient volume is inadequate to secure good prices in insurance and purchasing. These hospitals cannot afford to continue operating inefficient laundries, data processing centers, laboratories, and other support services. As a result, some administrators are sharing institutional services and are merging the operations of their hospitals with those of other hospitals on a regional basis, to improve economy of scale and to attract better management and technical support.

There are two models of such sharing:

1. *The multi-institutional system* provides the rural hospital administrator with opportunities for improved salary benefits, improved career mobility, and access to a greater variety of skills and experts.[3] These opportunities promote the possibility of operating efficiencies and better quality patient care.

Multihospital systems include the large for profit chains, the church-sponsored nonprofit system, the large nonprofit voluntary systems, and an assortment of small proprietary and nonprofit systems that tend to operate on a regional basis. The rural hospitals are affiliating with these systems through shared service arrangements, management contracts, lease agreements, and outright sales of these systems.

2. *Shared service programs* sponsored by aggressive state hospital associations are also increasingly available to rural hospitals whose governing boards and management prefer not to surrender as much autonomy. The close working relationship of the rural hospital administrator with governing board members, physicians, employees, patients, and visitors requires a management style that is often a bit more paternalistic than that found in larger institutions.

The rural hospital administrator has full management responsibility for all aspects of the hospital's operations, including financial management, personnel management, medical-legal affairs, patient care quality, and physical facilities management.

The rural hospital administrator performs in a glass house. Hard work and a creative approach to management are essential. Consumers, insurance companies, and governments join in applying pressure on rural hospital administrators to contain hospital costs in the face of an inflationary economy and an expensive medical technology. Like the urban hospital colleague, the rural hospital administrator confronts money shortages. Unlike many urban colleagues, the rural hospital administrator worries more about an inadequate supply of trained, competent personnel,[4] inadequate equipment that fails to meet the needs of local physicians, and suboptimal facilities that fail to meet advancing requirements for licensure, accreditation, and governmental life safety codes.

The rural hospital administrator is sought after to assume leadership positions in a wide variety of local civic and community activities, often enjoying close personal ties with the faculty of the state university medical school, with members of the state legislature and other agencies of state government, and with other leaders in various fields throughout a large regional area.

The rural hospital is increasingly extending itself outside its traditional four walls to address the new health needs perceived by the community. Imaginative administrators have led their governing boards and staff into such innovative ventures as physician office buildings, physician practice managements, prepaid health maintenance organizations, outreach clinics for isolated outlying towns, preventive health and health education programs, and facilities for improved health care for the elderly.

Some rural hospital administrators have concluded that the rural hospital is in the most strategic locus to own and operate a rural HMO.[5] One such example is that established by the Penobscot Bay Medical Center of Rockport, Maine, with the support, involvement, and cooperation of the local county medical society. Shortly after its inception, this venture had enrolled 2,300 persons on a prepaid basis, including low income persons whose premium payments were partially provided by federal health programs for the poor and the elderly.

Another example is the cooperative venture shared among the Garfield Memorial Hospital of Panguitch, Utah, and three local physicians serving that area. With the support and encouragement of the board, the medical staff, and the multihospital institution that manages this 17-bed county hospital under contract, the administrator has directed the development of three outlying ambulatory clinics and a rural home health care program for the elderly in the area. The one clinic houses three physicians adjacent to the hospital itself, while the other two are located as far as 70 miles away in Circleville and Escalante, Utah. These two communities had previously lacked immediate access to needed health care. In developing ambulatory care and home health services programs, the administrator faced major obstacles in obtaining working capital, personnel, and equipment. He or she solved the problems and derived enormous satisfaction from satisfying unmet health care needs.

Rural Medical Group Practice Management

The staff of the research division of the Medical Group Management Association of Denver, Colorado, estimates that at least 25 percent of their current 2,400 members work in rural settings of communities with 10,000 population or less.

Young physicians soon feel themselves ill equipped to handle their business management problems, and seek consultative assistance to manage the business aspects of their practice, and often their personal business as well. The entrepreneurial tradition that once motivated physicians is diminishing.[6] Young physicians entering rural practice increasingly seek partnerships, small corporations, or other forms of organizational arrangements that involve several physicians. These groups may be single specialty or multiple specialty. The evidence suggests that the long-term trend in which few physicians entered rural practice is being reversed.

As more of these multiphysician group practices are formed, the need for trained management to assist with their management responsibilities is also increasing. As with rural hospital administration, in the early days these management positions attracted people who were neither prepared nor experienced in management. People who had but modest training and experience in basic bookkeeping took these jobs as the group practices evolved. The growing complexity of managerial roles in rural group practice mirrors the growing complexity of third-party reimbursement programs and detailed tax laws.

The rural medical group manager oversees all aspects of the clinic's operation, including systems in admissions, medical records, business office management, and fiscal, personnel, and facilities management. The rural group practice manager must personify the work ethic and be a self-starter. The rural medical group manager manages fewer people and resources than the rural hospital administrator, but his or her responsibilities are no less challenging. (For a profile of the medical group practice administrator, see chapter 6.)

Physicians control and hire the rural medical group practice manager, who is usually a professional with demonstrated experience and defensible educational credentials. Here, the preferred educational discipline seems to be business administration. The more general the MBA pathway in business, the better. While also appropriate for rural medical group management positions, hospital or health administration degree graduates tend to be better oriented to nonprofit organizations and to larger institutional settings than to these small profit-oriented medical group practice management organizations.

Jobs in rural group practices are harder to locate because university facilities in the business schools do not keep files on them. The national professional organizations mentioned earlier will usually have information about openings. Occasionally ads are placed in national medical journals. Some medical groups contract with the professional medical recruiting and placement organizations. One of the better sources of information is the local medical group managers themselves.

Salary and fringe benefits for rural medical group managers vary widely. Physicians may initially have trouble assessing the capabilities of the new incumbent and, therefore, find it hard to judge the incumbent's worth. (This situation is explained in more detail in chapter 6.) Moreover, medical groups tend to survey the marketplace less skillfully than hospital boards customarily do.

Career patterns vary in rural group practice. Rural medical group managers tend to have very satisfying careers, and there is relatively little turnover in these jobs. In recent years, the Medical Group Management Association has operated a placement service and has usually averaged two to three dozen vacancies for these types of positions.

Some rural medical groups, particularly the smaller ones, are willing to hire managers without extensive experience. Some larger group practice managers have positions available for assistants. These can be excellent posts, particularly for providing the training and perspective useful for taking major management roles in the future. The Medical Group Management Association will sometimes broker a traineeship or preceptorship for a short period of time with a manager. The association can help you to locate these tailor-made training experiences, where the greatest amount of training and perspective can be gained in the shortest time. These are almost always in well-established group practice settings, where effective management systems are established, and where a veteran medical group manager is able and willing to serve as preceptor.

Rural medical group managers often will start their careers in smaller groups, and will either assist the organizations to grow, or move to progressively larger groups that operate on the scale with which they feel comfortable. On the other hand, many excellent managers prefer smaller groups and spend their entire careers in these organizations.

As with any career, there are factors that reflect both the satisfactions and the frustrations of the job. One major source of satisfaction with rural medical group practice management is that of working in a small-scale environment that is enjoyable to manage. In many cases warm satisfying interpersonal relationships develop, leading to high levels of mutual confidence among the principal physicians and the employees. Moreover, physicians are usually willing to recognize the worth of good management experience, and salary levels usually reflect increases commensurate with satisfactory performance. Frequently managers whose worth is recognized become part owners in the group practice with an opportunity to share in profits.

Still another source of the manager's satisfaction is that of providing leadership in the management of the investment portfolio of the group or of individual physicians. This responsibility can be a challenge in real estate, stocks, bonds, and other areas requiring sound investment. These latter opportunities become available particularly when the internal management systems and practices essential to efficient and effective clinic operation are functioning well.

Rural clinic managers find substantial satisfaction in directing and planning constructive projects to expand or replace the clinic's physical facilities. As in rural hospital administration, creative thinkers and doers are called for to assist their groups with such innovative ideas as establishing satellite clinic operations or diversifying toward other health related activities and organizations that fill hitherto unmet community health needs.

Major frustrations may develop as a result of the somewhat delicate relationship that must be maintained with the physicians who are the owners of the practice. Physician owners set the policies. Unlike the rural hospital's governing policy board, these policymakers may lack a breadth of interest, and they may be preoccupied primarily with achieving their goals on the bottom line of the profit and loss statement. Physicians have become much more concerned about their pricing structure and are applying increasing pressures on their managers to hold costs down. Efforts to improve efficiency and lower the group overhead can produce an ambiance of stress in the group practice as health care costs continue to rise.

Other Rural Health Administration Careers

Rural Health Planners

In early 1974 Cogress enacted the National Health Planning and Resources Development Act (Public Law 93–641), which became effective in January of 1975. This legislation establishes statewide agencies, as well as large areawide and subarea council planning organizations.[7] As this legislation came forth, many positions came into being in planning agencies where there had been a shortage of adequate, trained personnel. Because we are currently in the process of moving toward full implementation of this new local planning program, it is hard to document how many health planning jobs are available, or where they will be. Although there are a substantial number of jobs in rural subarea councils, the specific numbers and the locations of many of the subarea council operations are still in flux because this legislation is so new.

Rural health planners should receive a broad education as undergraduates, with substantial emphasis in the social sciences and statistics. Subsequent graduate training in public health administration and health planning is preferred.

Rural health planning involves developing profiles on community health characteristics and resources, forecasting health manpower and need projecting, analyzing and determining community health need requirements, and carrying out cost-benefit analysis.[8]

The subarea council health planner works under the direction of both the planning staff of state and areawide agencies and a local advisory board made up of community citizens who represent numerous social, economic, and racial consumer and health provider groups. The subarea health planner determines what health programs and resources are most appropriate to serve the consumers' needs in the given area. The subarea council provides supportable data and recommendations to the state and regionwide agencies upon which final decisions can be made about new programs and facilities.

The subarea council health planner's authority is limited mainly to a staff role, and he or she will often be caught up in heavy politics between diverse constituencies.

Rural Public Health Administration

Rural health administration is found in rural single county or multicounty public health departments. The trend for local county governments to form multicounty health department ventures calls for able, well-trained administrators. Qualifications for those administrators usually include a bachelor's degree in business or a closely related field, along with some accounting and economics. In most of these agencies there is a clear-cut preference for persons who have a master's degree in public administration. Rural public health administrators manage and coordinate programs and health personnel in a wide spectrum of health activities, including health care delivery, planning, facilities, licensure, public health education and counseling, and sanitation. These administrators are responsible for developing and managing the department's financial budgets. The responsibility for facilities management, program development, and much of the business activity is vested in or shared with others.

Most of these jobs are civil service jobs, with adequate but not overly generous remuneration. Political problems can be a major source of frustration because these local agencies operate under elected policy making officials and must coordinate or even be directed by statewide government health department agencies. The local health administrator can call on the expertise of the larger agencies to assist with complex technical problems. Rural public health administrators must be skillful in writing and in grantsmanship in order to secure state, federal, and private foundation funds to supplement their official tax-supported budgets. The directors of state public health departments and the faculties of schools of public health are the best sources of information on these positions.

Rural Nursing Home Administration

Rural nursing homes may be operated by either private individuals or private nursing home chain corporations. Other rural nursing homes may be sponsored by local governments. The privately run organizations are generally operated on a for profit basis, and many owners have sought to upgrade the quality of their managements in recent years. The best career opportunities appear to be with the multiple nursing home chains because they provide a better professional climate in which to work, better salary and benefits, and more opportunity for upward advancement based on satisfactory performance. Rural nursing home management may have less appeal to some because the consumers are the chronically ill and the aged. However, many capable managers have found substantial satisfaction in rural nursing homes because of the indispensable function they fill.

Here again, the emphasis is on attracting administrators with skills and experience in finance, facilities management, personnel, administration, health care reimbursement, data processing, etc. As a result, a few graduate university programs in hospital administration have developed special training pathways in nursing home management. In some cases, the well-established nursing home chains will aggressively recruit able people with backgrounds in nursing, business, and social services, and then provide the needed on-the-job training and experience necessary to qualify them as able administrators.

The rural nursing home administrator differs somewhat from other rural health administrators. Because of the kind of care provided in rural acute care general hospitals, the manager in a nursing home is less intensely involved with physicians. Indeed, the nursing home managers must assert themselves to persuade physicians to see their patients more frequently and to review the prescribed therapies. In addition, rural nursing homes generally do not operate laboratory, radiology, or other costly clinical support facilities. Patients who need these services are referred to acute care hospitals or to the doctor's office. Administrators concern themselves with support program areas such as food service, physical and occupational therapy, recreational therapy, and social activities.

Persons interested in rural nursing home administration should be aware that nursing home owners differ in their administrative philosophies. Some are idealistic and give generously of themselves in providing care for the old, the chronically ill, and the helpless who have been assigned to them. Others, regrettably, are instead oriented to the profit motive rather than to the care needs of patients. Some nursing homes are too small to be able to attract and support good management. Some of these operate in grossly inadequate facilities and without proper financial resources as well. On the other hand, many of the larger ones are developing excellent reputations, and they are succeeding in maintaining high public confidence by providing excellent health care for local residents who want to stay as close to home and family as possible.

In order to learn about specific opportunities in rural nursing home administration, it is advisable to check with state and national nursing home administrator organizations, large nursing home chains, professional medical personnel recruiting and placement agencies, and ads placed in national nursing home trade journals.

Salaries and benefits vary according to the size and complexity of the responsibility and the type of ownership. Nursing home managers are obliged now under federal mandate to undergo state licensure. Specific requirements are established in each state. In most cases an examination is required, and evidence of appropriate education and/or experience is also required. The professional nursing home administrator associations at both the state and the national levels can provide additional information on the implications of licensure and also offer assistance to candidates preparing for licensure.

Rural Mental Health Administration

Most rural mental health institutions are operated by state government, although a few are run by private organizations. In the western states most of the traditionally large state-owned mental hospitals are situated in small rural communities.

Individuals with both undergraduate and graduate degrees in business and hospital administration have taken responsible administrative jobs in these organizations. Those seeking positions in privately owned rural mental health institutions should be alert to factors similar to those mentioned earlier in nursing homes.

Administrative posts in state institutions are tied closely to civil service. In years past these jobs have usually been occupied by trained senior physicians, generally psychiatrists. However, administrative posts have passed to nonphysician health administrators because of the need for individuals with business skills and experience. Areas of major responsibility in these institutions include fiscal management, personnel administration, systems management, facilities management, medical-legal affairs, and many other related management areas. The state-operated institutions are often large enough to accommodate vertical career development. Some are relatively short and dead ended.

Policy is heavily influenced by elected public officials, and this often adds a certain amount of frustration to the rural mental health administrator's role. Local management is usually accountable to a department of state government headed by someone who is in turn accountable to the governor of the state. Candidates for positions often have to undergo civil service examination procedures prescribed by state law. Openings are generally best known by practicing administrators and state personnel agencies, although the trade journals and professional recruiting services may be useful. Salary and fringe benefits are generally adequate under provisions typical of state civil service programs.

In these assignments, the manager deals with physicians whose specialty is psychiatry. These institutions have a lesser emphasis on such acute health care services as laboratory, radiology, and other acute clinical support services. However, some of the large state mental institutions with large patient populations operate their own acute care hospitals as an integral part of their programs. In general, the main administrative emphasis is on good food and hotel services, occupational and recreational therapy, and individual and group psychotherapy.

Factors to Consider in Rural Health Administration

I shall identify some of the negative factors, as well as the positive factors, that generally apply to the rural health scene.

Virtually all rural health administration roles are subject to the following constraints:

1. insufficient number of physicians in rural areas
2. maldistribution and insufficient number of allied health personnel
3. inadequate access for consumers to health facilities and programs
4. lack of insurance coverage for poverty or near poverty levels among consumer groups
5. government intervention with universal solutions to complex problems that often require unique local prescriptions

6. heavy fluctuation in utilization patterns due to small-volume rural health operations which must support high fixed costs
7. some rural health consumers' ignorance of good health care
8. interrelationships with board members or other policymakers who may be somewhat uninformed and overly conservative.

But there are optimistic trends as well. Among these are the following:

1. development of educational shared service and referral linkages between small rural health organizations and their larger city regional and university medical center counterparts
2. newly trained types of personnel to fill gap areas, such as physician assistants, nurse practitioners, and paramedics
3. rural hospital outreach and new program developments, such as satellite clinics and community health centers, HMOs, home health programs, etc.
4. advent of rural multihospital and nursing home corporate systems and development of shared service arrangements
5. interest by national and state policymakers in the need for adequate rural health with renewed efforts to solve persistent problems
6. investment by medical schools and postgraduate medical training programs in family practice training for new physicians entering practice
7. increased interest by rural health consumers in becoming involved to assure that they have access to the care they desire and need.

Increasingly fewer people work in agricultural pursuits. Yet there appears to be a plateau effect, and in some instances a reversal, of the long-term pattern of people leaving the rural areas for the cities and the suburbs. The population growth that is now recurring in rural areas is expected to continue for many years.

Many rural communities and their health organizations are so small that the health administrator must perform several roles. For example, the rural hospital administrator in St. Anthony, Idaho, serves as the hospital administrator, the county coroner, the county ambulance driver, and the manager of a five-physician clinic. When he initially arrived on this job, he also had the responsibility for serving as the community's only laboratory and x-ray technician. Initially, the only formal college training he had was in these latter technical areas. In recent years, he has had the opportunity to acquire graduate training in hospital administration on a part-time basis, and he has had the opportunity to draw upon the expertise of a multihospital system. As a result, the level of his management performance and the satisfaction he receives therefrom have both increased substantially.

No two rural communities are alike—not even neighboring towns in the same county. Rural settings exist in almost every state in the nation, with the possible exception of small, densely populated states such as Rhode Island and Delaware. In states such as Wyoming, Idaho, Montana, and the Dakotas, virtually every community is rural. Some rural communities are fairly close to urban centers, making it possible to maintain the professional and cultural links essential to the needs of some who go into rural health administration.

There is the problem of taking a spouse into a rural community where the lifestyle is foreign to anything that person may have experienced before. People who are accustomed to such cultural activities as the theater, the symphony, art galleries, or the university, or people who are accustomed to enjoying major professional sports, may have a difficult time adjusting to rural life.

There is also the problem of gaining acceptance into a rural community where civic and social affairs are dominated by individuals from families that have been on the scene for many generations. The talented health administrator with a track record of worthy accomplishments can still be considered an outsider by people who have influence in the rural community.

There is also the factor of limited mobility. If for some reason he or she is unable to survive in a given job, the administrator may have difficulty finding suitable alternatives; these offerings are often remotely located.

Many rural communities have relatively homogeneous moral and ethical values. It is prudent to assess the cultural values of the local community before moving there. In the rural areas, incompatibilities can be devastating in both professional and private life. In these smaller communities news and gossip travel fast. High ethical standards and commitment to hard work and community activities are essential in most rural settings.

The Politics and Ethics of Rural Health Administration

Many major pieces of health legislation and their attendant regulations seem often not to provide for the special circumstances of rural health. As a result, the heavy hand of government bureaucratic regulation has given rise to considerable tumult in rural health organizations.

Prescriptions for the best therapies for the ills of rural health have continually been forthcoming from national health policy leaders and the government regulators alike, many of whom have virtually no basis for proper judgments.[9] Rural health organizations are mobilizing themselves politically. With the assistance of state and regional health professional associations, more rural health administrators are achieving more influential roles in political action at both the state and national levels. For many years the health industry was exempted from union activity under special provisions provided under national labor relations legislation. As these exemptions have been lifted, organized labor has initially concentrated its efforts on the major health organizations in large cities and industrial centers, and, as yet, the rural areas have been spared most of the attendant challenges and frustrations. Aggressive managements are taking preventive steps by elevating wage and benefit programs for employees commensurate with those in their neighboring urban areas.

In rural areas, different roles require different individuals with varying kinds of preparation. As the population continues to increase in rural America, health programs will grow and diversify. There will be more, rather than fewer, opportunities for administrators in rural health. Many well-trained and dedicated individuals who have recently taken positions in the rural health field are receiving tremendous satisfaction from their work. In the future, more will join them.

NOTES

[1] American Hospital Association, *Hospital Statistics* (1977 ed.). Chicago: American Hospital Association, 1977.

[2] Richard L. Johnson, "Rural Hospitals Face Change for a Bright Future." *Hospitals* 52, 2 (January 16, 1978):47.

[3] Donald C. Wegmiller, "Multi-Institutional Pacts Offer Rural Hospitals Do-or-Die Options." *Hospitals* 52, 2 (January 16, 1978):51.

[4] Verlyn Foster, "Should Small Hospitals Contract for Specialty Services?" *Hospitals* 48, (October 1, 1974):93.

[5] John R. Wheeler and Jefferson D. Ackor, "Should Small Hospitals Operate HMOs?" *Hospitals* 48, 19 (October 1, 1974):93.

[6] American Hospital Association, *Delivery of Health Care in Rural America.* Chicago: American Hospital Association, 1977.

[7]Steven Sieverts, *Health Planning Issues and Public Law 93-641*. Chicago: American Hospital Association, 1977.

[8]David F. Bergwall, Philip N. Reeves, and Nina B. Woodside, *Introduction to Health Planning*, Washington, D.C.: Information Resources Press, 1979.

[9]Robert L. Kane and Paul F. Westover, "Rural Health Care Research: Past Accomplishments and Future Challenges," *Transcultural Health Care Issues and Conditions*. Madeleine Leininger, ed. Santa Cruz, California: Davis Publishing Company, 1976. p. 123.

8 The Epidemiologist as Health Administrator

Pascal James Imperato, M.D., M.P.H. and T.M.

At a moment when at least verbal allegiance to quantitative decision making is fashionable among managers, it ought to be obvious that the quantitator par excellence—the epidemiologist—makes an indispensable contribution to health administration. Yet, the epidemiologist characteristically has been remote from health administrators' strategic decision making. This may have been due in part to efforts on the part of the old breed of physician epidemiologists in cooperation with old breed health administrators to keep it that way.

Pascal James Imperato, a career epidemiologist, has served as Health Commissioner of New York City. He tapped and applied his epidemiological skills and experience to his responsibilities as manager of a multimillion dollar public health agency. As non-M.D. epidemiologists in the future replace M.D. epidemiologists, they, too, are likely to pay a more prominent role in health administration. (L.E.B.)

The word "epidemiology" is derived from Greek roots and, narrowly defined, means "upon the people." A broader definition of the term applies to "the study of the distribution and dynamics of diseases in human populations."[1] Although epidemiology and its methods as we now know them have their roots in very ancient traditions of observation and reasoning, the term epidemiology did not come into use until the past century. In 1850 the Epidemiological Society of London was organized, and in 1873 the term epidemiology appeared in the title of a book, John Parkin's *Epidemiology; Or The Remote Cause of Epidemic Diseases In The Animal and In The Vegetable Creation.*[2]

During the latter half of the nineteenth century, and into the early decades of the present century, the prime focus of epidemiology was on the investigation of epidemic communicable diseases. The investigation of epidemics and the elucidation of such basic scientific concepts as mode of transmission, incubation period, period of communicability, susceptibility, resistance, and immunity progressed along with advances in the microbiological sciences. Even before the remarkable bacteriological advances of the late nineteenth century were made, physicians like John Snow had demonstrated how sophisticated investigational techniques could elucidate the sources and spread of communicable diseases. Snow's studies of cholera in London, published between 1850 and 1854, are epidemiologic classics, as are the studies of William Budd, who elucidated the epidemiology of typhoid fever in Bristol, England (1859–1860), and those of the Danish physician Peter Panum, who described measles in the Faroe Islands in 1846.

By the end of the nineteenth century, the mold of epidemiology was fairly well set. Its practitioners, although not called epidemiologists, investigated and controlled epidemics of communicable diseases. One could make a strong argument that at this

---

Pascal James Imperato, M.D., M.P.H., and T.M. is former Commissioner of Health for the City of New York. Currently, he is Professor and Chairman of the Department of Preventive Medicine and Community Health, State University of New York, Downstate Medical Center.

historical point epidemiology was primarily a methodology enmeshed in the broader area of sanitation. As the sciences of bacteriology and pathology developed, so did epidemiology. But it was viewed as a science rather restricted to the study of epidemics.[3]

The first attempt to broaden the focus of epidemiology came in the early part of this century under the impetus of William Welch. In effect, he said that epidemiology focused not only on disease epidemics, but also on the natural history of diseases, which included epidemics, endemics, and chronic infections. Although Welch thus broadened the concept of what epidemiology was concerned with, its focus remained on communicable diseases. But his ideas set the stage for expanding epidemiologic methods and for making epidemiology a deductive science. Attention was then given to the correlation of long-term disease trends; seasonal, host, and environmental factors; and the social determinants of disease.[4]

Epidemiology became institutionalized during the First World War and shortly thereafter at the federal, state, and city levels. An important step in the development of epidemiology as a scientific discipline and a medical specialty was the establishment of a Department of Epidemiology at the new Johns Hopkins School of Hygiene and Public Health in 1918. Wade Hampton Frost, by then one of the most outstanding epidemiologists in the United States, was asked to head the new department.[5]

In 1927 the American Epidemiological Society was founded, and there were many illustrious men among its charter members. Most of these men, and, indeed, most of those who were members of the Society in its early years were communicable disease epidemiologists, reflecting the Society's traditional focus and that of epidemiology in general.[6] However, by the 1950s, the membership of this Society had become quite heterogeneous, reflecting major shifts in disease trends. With the advent of antibiotics and the widespread use of both viral and bacterial vaccines, the incidence of most of the major communicable diseases fell dramatically in the United States. Cancer, heart disease, mental illness, accidents, and stroke soon headed the list of leading causes of death in the United States—ahead of any of the communicable diseases.

Many epidemiologists, based in teaching institutions and in federal government units, began to shift their attention away from the communicable diseases and towards the noncommunicable ones. But a substantial number of epidemiologists, particularly those attached to state and city health departments, remained deeply involved in communicable disease epidemiology, since it was an essential public health service. Even though the American Epidemiological Society had shifted much of its focus towards noninfectious diseases, by 1971 two-thirds of the papers presented at the annual meeting dealt with infectious diseases, reflecting the still strong commitment of many epidemiologists to the study of infectious diseases.[7]

Dilemmas of Epidemiologists Today

Epidemiology in the United States and elsewhere is deeply rooted in a long history of investigating and controlling communicable diseases. But the communicable diseases are no longer a paramount problem in the United States. The steady decline in the incidence of the major communicable diseases over the past two decades has made communicable disease epidemiology increasingly unattractive as a career to medical school graduates. Thus, fewer physicians enter the field each year, and the pool of existing physician-epidemiologists shrinks from attrition.

Logic would counsel the epidemiologic establishment to shift a significant level of its resources to chronic disease epidemiology and to health services planning, evaluation, and administration. But logic has not prevailed so far, for a number of complex reasons.

Within the past few years legislation has been enacted in Washington establishing Health Systems Agencies (HSAs), Professional Standards Review Organizations (PSROs), and laws governing health manpower, health services research, and health statistics. There is a need for more epidemiologists and for the incorporation of epidemiological concepts into all of these major areas affecting health care. Even if epidemiologists were willing to shift into these much needed areas, it is doubtful that they could do so, given the structure of our present health care system. In my view, major structural changes will have to take place in the health care system in the United States before this change can occur to a significant degree.

Epidemiologists who are unwilling to alter their present orientation towards the control of communicable diseases find themselves in a defensive posture in order to maintain budgetary supports for their activities. At the same time health care administrators and planners in dire need of epidemiologic expertise cannot find it.

Tyroler has pointed out that in the past 20 years epidemiologists in both the United States and Europe, seeking a separate professional identity, have developed elitist cliques.[8] Unwilling themselves to practice their discipline in the areas of health care planning, administration, and evaluation, they have also been unwilling to teach others how to practice it.

The exciting future of epidemiology in the United States lies in the areas of health care planning, evaluation, and administration. Physician-epidemiologists, who form the nuclei of these elitist cliques, are a vanishing breed. It is unlikely that they will discover new means for meeting future needs for epidemiologic expertise in health care administration. In the view of some, these needs may have to be met either by an entirely new breed of epidemiologist or by other individuals trained in epidemiologic techniques.

Physician Epidemiologists

The term epidemiologist covers a heterogeneous group of individuals whose training, functions, and organizational loci vary greatly in the United States. To this diverse group must be added those who, by reason of either training or experience, or both, possess epidemiologic skills and contribute some or most of their time to the management or administration of research and disease control programs.

Thus far, the focus in this discussion has been on physician epidemiologists, also known as medical epidemiologists. While a number of physicians are trained in postgraduate programs as epidemiologists in medical schools and schools of public health, the vast majority of physicians who enter the field do so through the Epidemic Intelligence Service of the U.S.P.H. Service Center for Disease Control. In February, 1975, Winkelstein surveyed all the schools of public health for the number of students who would graduate that year with doctoral degrees in epidemiology.[9] He found that the total number of physicians graduating was 14, and of nonphysicians, 21.

Under the impetus of the introduction of management and evaluation techniques into health care organizations, a number of schools of medicine have developed residency training programs designed to produce physicians who will be able to bring both management and epidemiological skills into clinical medicine. In 1975, Henderson surveyed schools of medicine for residency programs in general preventive medicine which included epidemiology as a significant component.[10] She found that 20 of the 26 general preventive medicine residency programs claimed to emphasize epidemiology and its application, 8 of the programs were in schools of medicine, 3 were jointly sponsored by schools of medicine and public health, 6 were in schools of public health, and 3 were in federal agencies. Of the 8, 6 medical school program directors stated that it was almost impossible to recruit graduating physicians into their program. The directors of the programs in the 6 schools of public health had more difficulty recruiting residents than did those in schools of medicine, and the 3 federal programs had few qualified applicants.[11]

Levit, Sabshin, and Mueller found that among the medical graduates of 1960, only 9 of 640 had chosen preventive medicine as their specialty.[12] Among the 1964 cohort, only 10 of 673 chose this specialty. It is estimated that only one in ten physicians who specialize in preventive medicine is an epidemiologist.[13] This means, therefore, that if present trends continue, physician epidemiologists will soon become a rarity.

To these small numbers of physician epidemiologists must be added the sizable number who are trained by the Epidemic Intelligence Service of the Center for Disease Control (CDC). At the present time the CDC annually recruits around 40 medical school graduates upon completion of their internships. During the period of the Vietnam War and the physician military draft, the CDC was able to recruit physicians quite easily into the Epidemic Intelligence Service. However, with the abolition of required military service for physicians, it has become increasingly difficult for them to recruit. The training program given to these physicians is known as the Epidemic Intelligence Service Training Course and consists primarily of several weeks of lectures and laboratory exercises covering general epidemiologic concepts and specific disease problems and biostatistics. The graduates of this course, known as Epidemic Intelligence Service Officers, are then given specific assignments for the remainder of their two-year tour of duty. A sizable number are assigned to local and state health departments, where they gain empirical training and experience primarily in communicable disease epidemiology under the guidance and supervision of state and city health department epidemiologists.

At the end of their tour, these physicians possess excellent experience in epidemiologic techniques and in the investigation and control of a large number of communicable diseases. In general, however, they function at a distance from the mainstream of administrative, evaluative, and managerial events in the organizational structures of which they are a part. As a consequence, they are not exposed to the larger vista of health care planning, evaluation, and administration. This is not a reflection of inadequacy on their part, but more a symptom of our present health care system, in which epidemiologic talent of this type is sequestered in a highly specialized categorical area.

Of the 691 physicians who graduated from the Epidemic Intelligence Service as of 1976 and who were not unemployed, retired, deceased, or lost to follow-up, 211 were in private practice or business, 42 were working in hospitals or like institutions, 39 were with state or local health departments, 9 were with other types of health agencies or groups, 91 were with the federal government, and 299 were associated with universities in various capacities.[14]

The career choices of the graduates of the Epidemic Intelligence Service are somewhat surprising. While 30.5 percent have gone into private practice or business, a significant number have remained in government, where many are presumably utilizing their epidemiologic skills.

A number of reasons explain why medical school graduates in the United States are not drawn into epidemiology as a career. As Henderson has stated, training centers in epidemiology are separated conceptually, physically, and professionally from medical students. Medical students are therefore unaware of career opportunities in epidemiology, and they have no role models to emulate. Epidemiology has low visibility in the clinical life of medical schools. This is due in part to a lack of awareness of its importance and usefulness by clinician professors who were trained in an era before epidemiology proved its usefulness in clinical medicine.[15]

Epidemiology is given a low priority in the curricula of most medical schools. The same can be said of general preventive medicine. In 1974, only 75 percent of the medical schools in the United States required a course in epidemiology.[16] Most advanced training programs in epidemiology are far removed from clinical settings which are viewed by medical students as having high status and value.

The potential earning capacity of a physician who currently chooses a career in epidemiology is small compared to someone who chooses a clinical specialty. What was once a disparity has now become a chasm, not only for epidemiologists but also for all those in preventive medicine. This earning difference commences in postgraduate training programs. Current high costs of medical education and the need of many medical school graduates to pay back loans or parents and relatives imposes high earning requirements on them as soon as they graduate. As Henderson has pointed out, the postdoctoral fellow in epidemiology or in a school of public health receives a stipend which is much lower than that of his or her clinical resident counterpart. The law of the marketplace drives physicians away from epidemiology.

Complicating this are the current income tax laws which favor the self-employed physician with a myriad of protective deductions, and penalize the salaried physician whose income receives no such relief from taxation. Seemingly attractive salaries no longer attract, since the net income scarcely suffices to support a modest middle-class existence. All of this results in an inability to recruit full-time physicians into epidemiology and preventive medicine in general.

Nonphysician Epidemiologists

Although highly trained and qualified individuals with other than M.D. degrees have chosen epidemiology as a career in past decades, their numbers were few. Only within the past two decades, and especially within the past few years, have nonphysicians chosen careers in epidemiology. Career opportunities for the nonphysicians have increased as physicians have progressively abandoned epidemiology. Hospitals and local and state health departments still face important day-to-day infectious disease problems which require management by well-trained professionals. In recent years they have come to rely increasingly on nonphysicians to provide these services. Nonphysician epidemiologists vary widely in terms of level and type of prior education, level and quality of training, and type of training and experience. This reflects both the absence of national and statewide guidelines, and also (and, perhaps, more importantly) the fact that in most instances, epidemiologists are trained individually for specific roles. For example, the functions of the epidemiologist who works in a hospital differ considerably from those of a public health counterpart who works in a local health department. Understandably, then, the level of recruitment, course content, and duration and level of training differ markedly.

Included among the nonphysician epidemiologists are those who are trained at the master's degree level, with or without any previous medical training; those who hold the bachelor's degree who have taken special nondegree courses of instruction in epidemiology; graduates of two and three year nursing school programs; paramedical personnel; and a number of others. The vast majority of these epidemiologists practice communicable disease epidemiology either in institutions or in public health departments. Only a minority, and primarily those with master's or doctoral degrees, are in research, or form part of academic faculties.

The terms nurse epidemiologist, lay epidemiologist, and hospital epidemiologist are commonly used today, as is the term infection control nurse. But those who fall under any one of these rubrics are heterogeneous in terms of overall training and experience, even within the same geographic area.

It is not unreasonable to assume that communicable disease epidemiology will be practiced in the future by nonphysicians. The New York City Department of Health, which has major communicable disease control responsibilities, began to suffer the progressive effects of physician attrition and an inability to recruit new staff members into its epidemiology program in the early 1960s.[17] New York City's case history illustrates not only the problem of staffing but also its solution. This solution is but one model; it may not be suitable in other communities. It warrants some detailed discussion, since it clearly exposes what is happening across the country.

The New York City Department of Health Epidemiology Program, 1900–Present

Epidemiologic activities have been carried out in New York City since the eighteenth century. It was not until the latter part of the nineteenth century that the Department of Health institutionalized these activities within the administrative framework of a Division of Contagious Diseases. A principal activity of this division, and of the organizations that replaced it, was the accurate clinical diagnosis of reported cases of communicable disease. Reports of specific communicable diseases were not accepted on their face value, especially in the years before accurate confirmatory laboratory tests were widely available. This meant that individual patients had to be examined by skilled and experienced diagnosticians and the diagnosis of the reporting physician either upheld or rejected on clinical grounds. Control measures hinged upon the confirmatory diagnosis; for this reason, the Department of Health developed a cadre of well-trained diagnostician-epidemiologists—clinical physicians with diagnostic acumen.

From the 1920s through the 1950s the Department of Health was able to recruit and retain sufficient numbers of physician-epidemiologists, especially during the years of the Great Depression, when the steady income of municipal employment was an inducement. After World War II, the older members of the staff remained, since they had a large investment in pensions. But it became increasingly difficult to recruit younger physicians because of the relatively low salaries offered by the department, compared to the potential remuneration of private practice and the incomes available in private and university employment.

In order to deal with the problem of recruitment, the Department's Bureau of Preventable Diseases came to rely increasingly on the services of part-time physicians who were paid for each session. Most of these physicians were pediatricians, internists, and general practitioners in private practice who worked an average of two and one-half hours per day for the Bureau of Preventable Diseases.

By the mid-1960s, many of the full-time medical epidemiologists who had entered the Department of Health in the 1930s began to retire. The responsibility for providing epidemiologic services devolved increasingly upon the part-time epidemiologists. This was a less than satisfactory situation, since many types of outbreak require long hours of field work. Part-time staff do not have the time to conduct such investigations properly. Between 1965 and 1974 most of the serious outbreaks were managed by a small nucleus of full-time staff who often served long overtime hours without remuneration.

In 1970, 31 part-time field epidemiologists were employed by the Department of Health. The Division of Epidemiology in which they worked was headed by a full-time medical epidemiologist and staffed with one full-time medical epidemiologist. In addition, the division provided experience and training to one epidemic intelligence service officer from the U.S. Public Health Service Center for Disease Control. The Chief of the Division of Epidemiology reported to a full-time medical Director of the Bureau of Infectious Disease Control.

By 1972, the Division of Epidemiology had lost both its chief and its remaining full-time epidemiologist, thereby causing an upward shift of operational responsibility to the Director of the Bureau of Infectious Disease Control. This person was also responsible for administering the Division of Tropical Medicine, which operates four clinics in the city and provides for 25,000 visits per year; the Division of Veterinary Medicine; and the Immunization Program.

In spite of intensive efforts, the Department was unable to attract any candidates for either the position of Chief Epidemiologist or the four full-time epidemiologist positions. There were several reasons for this inability to recruit. Salary levels were locked into the New York City civil service system and were about 25 percent less than those for comparable positions in state and national governments. Even with parity salaries, it is difficult to attract professionals into New York City because of the relatively high cost of living and the high state and city income taxes.

In 1970, the field epidemiology program was costing the Department of Health an average of $444,000 per year. The part-time services provided were mainly routine case investigations of hepatitis, salmonellosis, and meningitis. Whenever there were outbreaks of other serious diseases such as trichinosis, diphtheria, and botulism, the small full-time staff had to take over, since the part-time epidemiologists could not manage these problems adequately during the two and one-half hours a day they were employed. In 1972, the routine investigation of cases of salmonellosis was discontinued.

TABLE 8-1

FIELD ACTIVITIES OF MEDICAL EPIDEMIOLOGISTS BY DISEASE AND BOROUGH, NEW YORK CITY, 1970

Borough	Total number of cases assigned for investigation	Hepatitis		Samonellosis		Meningitis		Other diseases	
		Number	Percent of total in borough	Number	Percent of total in borough	Number	Percent of total in borough	Number	Percent of total in borough
Bronx	1,685	496	30	403	24	442	26	344	20
Brooklyn	2,292	1,196	52	517	23	187	8	392	17
Manhattan	1,934	950	49	399	21	379	19	206	11
Queens	1,268	788	62	143	11	107	9	230	18
Richmond	454	371	82	26	6	24	5	33	7
Totals	7,633	3,801	50	1,488	19	1,139	15	1,205	16

Source: Author's data.

Up to that time, cases usually were investigated on the basis of a reported positive stool culture. Such reports did not reach the department until a week or more after the illness. Consequently, these routine investigations were rarely profitable from an epidemiologic point of view. Since 1972, only certain outbreaks or clusters of cases have been investigated. This change in policy reduced the case load of field epidemiologists by almost 20 percent. Their routine investigations of hepatitis, meningitis, and other diseases produced mainly case-specific clinical details, but little or no epidemiologic data. In 1974, the Department of Health modified its antirabies treatment policy in order to bring it into line with known epidemiologic data, and this greatly reduced the need for antirabies clinics and for epidemiologists to staff them.

Because of these facts, the program's cost, its poor adaptation to existing needs, and the Department's inability to recruit personnel, it was decided to establish a new program staffed by full-time public health nurse-epidemiologists.

Selection of Nurses for Program

All candidates were registered professional nurses, graduates of approved baccalaureate nursing programs, who were licensed to practice in the United States. The candidates were recruited exclusively from among the 460 public health nurses then working in the Department of Health's Bureau of Public Health Nursing. The skills acquired by public health nurses who work in the Department of Health's district health centers and clinics, and the specific experiences they have from various epidemiologic field investigations throughout the city, provide them with an excellent background for training as public health epidemiologists. The ten candidates who were selected had an average of 4.01 years (median 2.83 years) of experience in public health nursing. In addition, all candidates were required to have some hospital experience. This provides the sound background in the medical, laboratory, administrative, and recording procedures of hospitals that is needed to investigate reports of infectious diseases. The average number of years of hospital-based nursing experience prior to entrance into public health nursing was 9.35 years (median 9.00 years). Selection was limited to public health nurses who had taken courses in microbiology, biostatistics, and epidemiology in nursing school, and who had received at least a B average in each of these subjects.

Finally, each candidate's work performance records were reviewed. Annual supervisor reports from the Bureau of Public Health Nursing were examined, special attention being given to punctuality, self-direction, competence in nursing practice, and motivation for continued learning. The final selection of the candidates was based on all of these qualifications.

The Nurse-Epidemiologist Training Program

The training program lasted 30 weeks; it began with 6 weeks of lectures, followed by 12 weeks of a closely supervised work-study (internship) experience, and concluded with 12 weeks of field work. The program was designed to build upon the nurses' background in public health so that they would become competent to perform the duties of public health epidemiologists that are listed in Table 8-2.

The initial six-week didactic period consisted of an intensive presentation of basic concepts which integrated lectures, problem-solving seminars, and discussion workshops based on the lectures. The course in biostatistics stressed the collection, tabulation, graphing, and comparison of vital statistics. The students were also introduced to elementary sampling techniques and life-expectancy tables. Great emphasis was placed on the development of the practical skills needed to interpret and present data effectively.

The course in epidemiology was divided into two equal segments. During the first three weeks the nurses were taught principles and methods of epidemiology. These included concepts of cause, patterns of disease occurrence, genetic and environmental

TABLE 8–2
DUTIES OF PUBLIC HEALTH NURSE-EPIDEMIOLOGISTS,
CITY OF NEW YORK DEPARTMENT OF HEALTH, 1975

(1) Provide information regarding the incidence, control, and prevention of infectious diseases to medical practitioners and the general public.
(2) Supervise and participate in epidemiological investigations to determine sources of infection or vehicles of transmission.
(3) Institute immediate control and preventive measures such as isolation of cases and immunization and quarantine of contacts in outbreaks of disease.
(4) Assist hospitals in the investigation and control of nosocomial infections.
(5) Coordinate outbreak-control measures with local health officials, hospital infection-control committees, and epidemiologists.
(6) Participate in the education of persons involved in the prevention of infectious disease.
(7) Serve as preceptors or role models in field practice for nursing and medical students.
(8) Act as consultants in epidemiology to other professional disciplines and the community.
(9) Conduct studies and investigations of public-health problems involving noncommunicable diseases and environmental hazards.

Source: Author.

determinants of disease, and methods of study (cohort, case control, clinical trials). The students also were introduced to screening, principles of immunization and chemoprophylaxis, and selected aspects of chronic and congenital disease. The second three-week period was an in-depth presentation of the epidemiology and importance to public health of specific infectious diseases that the public health epidemiologists might encounter during their future assignments.

The course in microbiology complemented the epidemiology of infectious diseases, in that the students became familiar with the laboratory techniques necessary to augment their epidemiologic investigations through lectures and practical experience. Students learned methods for microbial sampling of the environment, respiratory infections, and food-borne and water-borne diseases. They reviewed basic concepts in the interpretation of bacteriologic, virologic, and serologic findings. Finally, they participated in survey exercises to familiarize themselves with the bacteriologic flora in the hospital environment and in the respiratory tract.

The course in environmental sanitation emphasized the roles of air, water, heating, ventilation, air conditioning, illumination, noise, and radiation in health-related problems. The students became familiar with the problems of pest control, animals, drugs, and toxins such as lead poisoning. They also learned principles of inspection, sampling, standards, and testing necessary to quantitate environmental hazards.

The course in administration and resources was oriented toward defining the role of the nurse-epidemiologist in New York City. The organization of health services on the city, state, and federal levels was described. The students also reviewed the New York City Health Code and the specific health forms and methods of collecting data and analyzing statistics that they would use.

The work-study experience was divided into three periods of four weeks each. Two periods were spent working under the supervision of a hospital nurse-epidemiologist. A total of four hospitals participated in the program; two students were assigned to one hospital for a four week period and then rotated to another hospital for a second four weeks. One day each week the students returned for a planned program of continuing education; this included lectures, seminars, tutorial sessions, case presentations, and field trips.

During this phase of the internship the students were exposed to the knowledge, skills, and attitudes of hospital nurse-epidemiologists and were able to gain an understanding of the problems inherent in dealing with hospital-associated infections and outbreaks. Under the direct supervision of hospital nurse-epidemiologists, students were given the opportunity to make rounds of nursing units for the purpose of case finding, to determine the suitability of procedures for isolation, to maintain records of patients with infections, to identify employee problems, and to teach others about infection control techniques and problems. In addition, the students were asked to help identify and investigate possible sources of infection within the hospital, report required diseases to the City of New York Department of Health, assist in developing the monthly report of infections, attend various meetings and conferences relevant to the control of infection, and be aware of environmental hazards (including problems concerning sterilization and disinfection).

The third four-week period was spent at the Department of Health's Bureau of Infectious Disease Control. Students observed the functioning of the Bureau's central office as reports of infectious disease were received, confirmed, tabulated, assigned, investigated, and completed. Toward the end of the four-week period, the students accompanied the full-time physician-epidemiologists in investigations of case reports or outbreaks of infectious diseases.

Throughout the twelve-week work study experience, one day each week was devoted to planned continuing education. Morning sessions included two segments of two hours each. The initial two-hour segment consisted of a critical analysis of a recent journal article dealing with an outbreak or epidemic of a disease.

Afternoon sessions consisted of field trips to various health agencies, including the Department of Health's Bureau of Laboratories, Poison Control Center, Medical Examiner's Office, Tropical Disease Clinics, and Restaurant Inspection Bureau, as well as a field trip to the Quarantine Center at Kennedy Airport. During these sessions the students were encouraged to ask questions about the mission of each agency and its relation to their future work.

Once their training program was completed, the nurse-epidemiologists were awarded conjoint diplomas from the New York City Department of Health and the Cornell University Medical Center–New York Hospital School of Nursing. They were then assigned to work full-time in one of five borough offices under the supervision of the Department's full-time central office staff and the part-time physicians who serve as borough chiefs.

Comparative Work Performance of the Nurse-Epidemiologist and the Part-Time Physician-Epidemiologist, 1975

To compare the work performance of the nurse-epidemiologists and the part-time physician-epidemiologists, a retrospective analysis of certain of their investigations was undertaken in December of 1975. This analysis was limited to investigation reports submitted by both groups on viral hepatitis and infections of the central nervous system. All reports of these two types of investigations submitted since January 1, 1975, were reviewed consecutively until 1,000 cases of viral hepatitis and 500 cases of central nervous system infections were collected. These reports represent approximately 90 percent and 95 percent, respectively, of the year's total number of cases for these two conditions.

Two parameters were examined in these reports, one quantitative and the other qualitative. The quantitative measure consisted of the average number of days between assignment of the case to an epidemiologist and submission of the final report. The qualitative measure consisted of the presence of comments on the report forms. Case reports often require some detailed comments in order to amplify the data that are coded on the investigation form. For the purpose of this analysis, case reports lacking such comments were considered to be inadequately completed. Case reports of viral hepatitis were also examined for information concerning whether the patient had been tested for hepatitis B antigen and whether the result was positive, negative, or pending.

As is shown in Table 8-3, the nurse-epidemiologists completed their investigations of cases of both viral hepatitis and central nervous system infections more quickly than the part-time physician-epidemiologists. The difference in the average number of days required for completion of cases of central nervous system infections is highly significant. There also is a highly significant difference between the physicians and the nurses in regard to comments on the case reports and the recording of data on hepatitis B antigen testing (P = <0.0001). In summary, the analysis revealed that nurse-epidemiologists completed their assignments more quickly and more efficiently than the part-time physician-epidemiologists. This allowed the Department to institute control measures more rapidly and more effectively.

Comparative Costs of the Epidemiology Programs

In 1975 the average per hour remuneration of the Department's part-time physician-epidemiologists was $19.05. The four physicians who served as part-time chiefs of epidemiology in the five boroughs are remunerated at the slightly higher rate of $21.45 per hour. The total cost of this program was $440,000 per year.

As of January 1, 1976, all of the part-time physician-epidemiologists were terminated except for the four borough chiefs and five physician-epidemiologists. The work performance of these nine part-time physician-epidemiologists consistently had been of higher quality than that of those who were terminated. This cadre and the full-time staff of the Bureau of Infectious Disease Control (renamed Bureau of Preventable Diseases on January 1, 1976) now provide the necessary medical backup to the nurse-epidemiologists. The total annual cost of the services of these nine physicians' time is $120,000.

The annual cost of the services of the Department's ten nurse-epidemiologists is $158,000. This, added to the cost of the part-time physician-epidemiologist services, totals $278,000 per year, or $162,000 less than the cost of the previous part-time physician-epidemiologist program. Thus, the Department of Health was able not only to improve considerably the quality and efficiency of its epidemiologic services with its new program but also to realize an annual saving of $162,000.[18]

The Implications of the New York City Nurse Epidemiology Program

New York City's epidemiology program is at present staffed by public health nurses, as I have described above, together with two nonphysicians with master's degree level training in epidemiology. They all work under the supervision of a nucleus of physician epidemiologists. Henderson has pointed out that while such professionals make enormous contributions to the management and administration of disease control programs, they play little or no role in the areas of policymaking and planning.[19] In other words, epidemiologists of this type are rather peripheral to the decision making that concerns major health planning, evaluation, and administration. Some would argue that this is not a deficiency, on the grounds that their services are crucial to a vital public health activity, and they cannot be spared for the broader vistas of planning, administration, and evaluation.

Most of the new training programs in epidemiology have been producing professionals who will manage disease control programs in either public health departments or in hospitals. Epidemiologists in educational centers such as schools of public health and departments of preventive medicine have remained rather isolated within their own disciplinary compounds and have had little or no impact on health services administration.[20] Gittlesohn has justifiably said that both epidemiologists and biostatisticians as a group, with few exceptions, have given little attention to the difficult problems of health services administration.[21] They have preferred to focus on studies involved with etiology, using methods and theories in controllable settings such as the laboratory and the clinic.

TABLE 8-3
COMPARATIVE WORK PERFORMANCE OF NURSE-EPIDEMIOLOGISTS AND PART-TIME PHYSICIAN-EPIDEMIOLOGISTS, CITY OF NEW YORK DEPARTMENT OF HEALTH, 1975

	Viral hepatitis				Central nervous system disorders		
	Number of reports	Average number of days to complete investigation	Reports with comments (percent)	Reports with comments on hepatitis B antigen (percent)	Number of reports	Average number of days to complete investigation	Reports with comments (percent)
Part-time physician-epidemiologists	776	7.95	51.4	13.2	304	22.6	54.7
Nurse-epidemiologists	224	7.40	98.8*	75.5*	196	7.30*	98.9*

Source: Author's data.
*P= <0.0001

Obviously, then, epidemiologists of both the old breed and the new remain isolated from the health services field. Most epidemiologists are not, in fact, linked in a meaningful way to policy planning and key decision-making processes in the health services field. In addition, most physician-epidemiologists in the public sector in the United States are not in key administrative positions and do not tend to move up in an organization from their disease control responsibilities into broader administrative roles. Many are not interested in making such career moves, and the few who are may not be perceived as having the competence to fill these different roles. Top health administrators in public health agencies tend to favor keeping the physician-epidemiologist where he or she is, since the upward movement into a more responsible administrative post would create a vacancy that would be hard to fill.

Those physician-epidemiologists who do assume important administrative positions in the broader health services field are more often individuals who have had some epidemiologic training as part of broader administrative training than they are pure physician-epidemiologists. In reality, they are physician-administrators with epidemiologic training and experience, and not physician-epidemiologists. The difference is an important one, and not so fine as one might think.

The Present Role of Epidemiologists in Health Administration

It is abundantly clear from what has been said so far that epidemiologists of all types in the United States currently have little or no role in health services planning, administration, and evaluation. At the risk of being repetitive, I can say that not only are epidemiologists not in key administrative positions, but also they and their skills are not meaningfully linked to those who are, or to the planning and administrative processes they control. True, epidemiologists in the public sector may manage and administer units in their given organizations, and those in the academic and institutional settings similarly may head units or departments. But this level of administration is a far cry from that involved in planning and evaluating broad health services programs.

The accrued experience of most epidemiologists tends to seem narrow, because we live in an era of broadening health services problems of which they have little or no knowledge. It is difficult for them, therefore, to shift over into this complex arena and to be useful there without some refurbishing. I vividly recall my shock when speaking with an eminent physician-epidemiologist in 1976 about the National Health Planning and Resources Act of 1974 (Public Law 93–641), which mandated the establishment of Health Systems Agencies (HSAs) throughout the country. He had heard of neither the law nor its implementation! My lengthy explanation of both and analysis of their implications for the future did not stir much interest on his part. Were such an anecdotal experience rare and isolated, it could be viewed as an irrelevant tidbit. Unfortunately, it is more the rule than the exception.

The public policy issues and problems embodied in the allocation of what are now known to be limited health care resources in the United States have been rendered more acute by the rapidly rising costs of health care, the presence of expensive duplicative technologies and services, the uneven distribution of resources and services, and the recognition that the quality of preventive, therapeutic, and diagnostic services is not always what it should be. As White has pointed out, there is an acute need in this country to bring to bear upon these problems the benefits of the quantitative approaches which epidemiology has to offer; these approaches are allied to those which demography, sociology, and public health statistics have to offer.[22] At present, neither epidemiologists nor epidemiology is doing the job, and they are not likely to do it as long as they remain cloistered in a closet of curiosities. Rare exceptions are those administrators who have had significant epidemiologic training and experience, and who are able to bring these to bear upon the broader health services problems with which they deal.

The Future Role of Epidemiologists in Health Administration

Most of the issues discussed so far have been of concern to health administrators, government officials, and epidemiologists for quite a few years. In 1975, the Health Resources Administration of the U.S. Department of Health, Education and Welfare sponsored a major important conference on the uses of epidemiology as a fundamental science in health services planning, administration, and evaluation. This conference was organized by the International Epidemiological Association, whose Council members participated in it.[23] Coming from different countries and from both governmental and academic settings, the participants were able to identify the problems and opportunities now facing epidemiology as a science and as an administrative tool. Endicott, in his Foreword to the Proceedings of this conference, points out the pivotal importance of epidemiologists and biostatisticians in our current and future health care delivery systems. He has stressed that decision-making processes and their outcomes can be greatly influenced by the knowledge and skills which epidemiology has to offer. And he goes on to say that the United States, with an annual health care expenditure of fifteen billion dollars, cannot afford the luxury of postponing the use of epidemiological and biostatistical methodologies and skills in dealing with health care problems.[24]

What is clear from all of the comments and discussions made during this conference is that epidemiologists are not currently playing the role they should in health care administration. What also emerged, and what has been known for a long time to the ˋcognoscenti, is that epidemiologists comprise a heterogeneous group of scientists. Reflecting this in part are the diverse applications of epidemiology: practical day-to-day public health communicable disease control, research in institutional settings, health services research focusing on program development and evaluation, and the role of epidemiology in relation to decision-making processes concerned with resource allocation and the organization of health services. In the latter two broad areas, there is currently a dearth of participation on the part of epidemiologists. Participants in this conference recognized, however, that not only are more epidemiologists of the traditional models needed, but also a new breed of epidemiologist who can combine his or her knowledge with the disciplines of economics, management sciences, political science, and public administration, and who will be part of a team which will include planners, administrators, and other decision makers. The major new future roles of the epidemiologist will be in health services research and in decision-making processes governing resource allocation and the organization of health services. How this is to come into being is currently a topic of intense discussion; it will require resolution rather soon if the new federal initiatives in health care planning and evaluation are to be adequately influenced by epidemiologists and their skills.[25]

Another area which is in crucial need of development is the teaching of epidemiologic principles and methods to health administrators. Allusion has already been made to the absence of formal training in epidemiology in a significant number of schools of public health in the United States.[26] The same situation—and worse—exists in schools of public administration, the spawning grounds of many current and future health administrators. Courses of an intensive nature would, in the short term, confer some epidemiologic expertise on health care administrators. In the long term, epidemiology should be an important and integral part of the formal training of every health care administrator.

The recruitment, training, placement, and development of long-term career lines and opportunities for epidemiologists in health care administration is a pressing need. But before this can happen, there must be structural changes in our health care system to provide a place for the country's new breed of epidemiologist. These changes are now taking place, and the dialogue has begun; the epidemiologist whose future will be in health care administration is even now in the making.

NOTES

[1] P.E. Sartwell, *Preventive Medicine and Public Health*. New York: Appleton-Century Croft, 1965.

[2] G. Rosen, "An Epidemiologist Views His Discipline." *Yale Journal of Biology and Medicine* 46, no. 1 (1973): pp. 1–2.

[3] F.G. Crookshank, "First Principles and Epidemiology," *Proceedings of the Royal Society of Medicine* 13 (1919–1920): pp. 159–84.

[4] J.R. Paul, "Historical Setting, An Account of the American Epidemiological Society—A Retrospect of Some Fifty Years." *Yale Journal of Biology and Medicine* 46, no. 1 (1973): pp. 5–14.

[5] *Ibid.*

[6] *Ibid.*

[7] *Ibid.*

[8] H.A. Tyroler, Discussion of paper, "Great Britain: A Strategy for Research and Training in Epidemiology," by E.G. Knox, in *Epidemiology as a Fundamental Science: Its Uses in Health Services Planning, Administration, and Evaluation*, ed. Kerr L. White and Maureen M. Henderson. New York: Oxford University Press, 1976.

[9] W. Winkelstein, as cited by M.M. Henderson in "Needs and Resources for Epidemiology as a Fundamental Science," in White and Henderson, *op. cit.*

[10] M.M. Henderson, "Needs and Resources for Epidemiology and Health Statistics in the United States," in White and Henderson, *op. cit.*

[11] *Ibid.*

[12] E.J. Levit, M. Sabshin, and C.B. Mueller, "Trends in Graduate Medical Education and Specialty Certification, A Tracking Study of United States Medical School Graduates," *New England Journal of Medicine* 290 (1974): pp. 545–49.

[13] M.M. Henderson, *op. cit.*

[14] Center for Disease Control, *Epidemic Intelligence Service 1976 Directory*. Atlanta: The Center, 1977

[15] M.M. Henderson, *op. cit.*

[16] W.H. Barker, "ATPM Survey," *Association of Teachers of Preventive Medicine Newsletter* 21, no. 1 (1974): pp. 10–14.

[17] P.J. Imperato, L.M. Drusin, J.S. Marr, E.C. Lambertsen, and B. Topf-Olstein, "The New York City Nurse Epidemiology Program," *Bulletin of the New York Academy of Medicine* 53, no. 6 (1977): pp. 569–85.

[18] *Ibid.*

[19] M.M. Henderson, *op. cit.*

[20] J.R. Evans, "Planning and Evolution in Canadian Health Policy and Programs," in White and Henderson, *op. cit.*

[21] A. Gittlesohn, Discussion of paper, "Canada: Epidemiology in the Planning Process in British Columbia, Description of an Experience with a New Model," by D.O. Anderson, in White and Henderson, *op. cit.*

[22] K.L. White, Preface to White and Henderson, *op. cit.*

[23]White and Henderson, *op. cit.*

[24]K.M. Endicott, Foreword to White and Henderson, *op. cit.*

[25]White and Henderson, *op. cit.*

[26]M.M. Henderson, *op. cit.*

9 As Emergency Medical Services Administrator

Barry A. Cooper, M.H.A.

Just as form follows function in modern architecture, so do specialties in health administration come into being in response to belatedly acknowledged needs that require an organized response. One of the latest examples of such specialties is emergency medical services (EMS). Health care emergencies have always been around, but it is only recently that they have been attended to by trained paraprofessionals and professionals working in complex communications and organizational networks.

Barry Cooper discusses how to improve the quality of EMS so that the intervention following biologic catastrophe is timely and of a quality to enhance the chances of the patient's restoration with minimal pathophysiologic damage. (L.E.B.)

Mainstream jobs in health administration include those of hospital administrator, health planner, long-term administrator, and public health administrator. However, the advent of new technologies, together with the participation of government in health affairs, has resulted in the establishment of health programs that focus on comparatively specific segments of the health system. These programs operate in highly specialized areas, such as end-stage renal disease networks, home health care programs, and Professional Standards Review Organization (PSRO) developments.[1] In this chapter we will look at the health administrator in one of these less well-known professional areas: emergency medical service (EMS) systems administration.

A personal, traumatic experience, or the less trying experience of a television drama may make the ordinary citizen aware of EMS. However, not everyone realizes the complexity and often the frustration of the work that is required to keep the sirens whining and the lights flashing. This chapter will show you what an EMS system is; how the EMS administrator helps, and occasionally hinders, the delivery of emergency medical services; and how you prepare to become an EMS administrator. In addition, it concerns system trends, the profession, the individual's role in shaping it, and the future impact of EMS systems administration. The following quotation sets the scene:

> *It has been projected that 18,000 accident victims out of the 115,000 who die annually might be saved if proper immediate care were rendered.*
> *Preventable pre-hospital coronary heart disease deaths have been conservatively estimated to number 50,000 per year.*
> *At least 5,000 of the deaths from other causes such as poisoning, drowning, obstetrical complications, etc., are deemed preventable.*
> Emergency Medical Services: Problems, Programs and Policies. *A statement prepared by the Committee on Public Policy of the American College of Emergency Physicians, 1977.*

Barry A. Cooper, M.H.A., is Senior Associate, American College of Preventive Medicine.

The EMS Systems Concept: Big Government and Local Initiative

The EMS systems administrator plans, organizes, implements, and evaluates. In concert with doctors, nurses, emergency medical technicians (EMTs), staff specialists, and the public, the administrator coordinates prehospital and hospital services designed to decrease morbidity and mortality caused by emergency illness.

A first aid course for the public, a phone call for help during a medical emergency, the treatment delivered at the scene of an accident, and the ambulance ride to the hospital belong to the prehospital phase of emergency medical care. The prehospital phase is complete when the patient arrives at the hospital emergency department. In the hospital phase, more comprehensive care is available. The patient may be treated at the emergency department and released, perhaps to return to a clinic or to a doctor's office for follow-up or rehabilitative care. The more seriously ill patient will be admitted to the hospital and rushed to the surgical suite for emergency surgery or to the intensive care unit (ICU) that is designed for the care of the critically ill inpatient. The emergency department will, generally, not treat the inpatient, but it is the department through which many are admitted to the hospital.

A long neglected area of health care delivery, EMS has undergone impressive development since the mid-nineteen-sixties. Few EMS system administrators existed before that time, and nobody was responsible for coordinating regional emergency care activities.

In 1965 the accident death toll in the United States was at an alarming 107,000, and it continued to rise. The quality of emergency medical services was a national disgrace. A description of Iowa's prehospital activities in 1968 is indicative:

> ...[Sixty percent] of ambulance services were run by undertakers. Of these only half required any first aid training at all of prospective employees, and 80% had no regular inservice training; 48% gave no first aid "in bad cases" before the patient was picked up, and 30% gave none at all, "because our business is transportation." Some 29% of all ambulances were more than 10 years old. About 60% carried no splints. Only 48% of the operators bothered to clean the medical equipment after each use. [2]

Lyle Shook, the study's director, commented, "These data for Iowa are little different from those gathered in other states. The picture of ambulance service is very discouraging."

Evidence of the improvement in prehospital care organization lies in the shift away from the funeral hearse ambulance service. In 1976, 60 percent of all ambulance services were operated by volunteer squads, 20 percent by municipal (e.g., fire department) services, 10 percent by hospital-based services, and 10 percent by commercial operators. [3] The undertakers, confronted with increasingly numerous requirements for more germane technological and management capabilities, could not survive in the new EMS systems. Few had the wherewithal to train their personnel to become EMTs as the government began to require. Fewer could afford to pay the increased salaries of the EMTs.

EMTs are new and valuable members of the EMS patient care team. They are particularly active in the prehospital phase, where they deliver life-saving care using an array of sophisticated procedures and equipment. EMTs are also contributing to hospital-based EMS delivery, representing but one of the new developments in the emergency department.

The emergency department, long thought to be an appendage of the hospital, has become increasingly more important in the total hospital organization. During the period from 1954 to 1973, emergency room visits have increased sixfold, growing more than any other hospital department during the same period. [4] In response to this unprecedented growth, the career emergency physician has emerged. The EMS specialist is replacing the on-call emergency physician, whose primary interests often lie in other specialized areas. Today, thousands of full-time emergency physicians are employed in the nation's hospitals. [5]

Formed in 1968, the American College of Emergency Physicians (ACEP) is in the process of setting up a new specialty board, the American Board of Emergency Medicine. Federally funded residencies in emergency medicine are coming into being throughout the country. A similar expansion of numbers is occurring among EMTs and nurses specializing in emergency care. The organization of the National Association of Emergency Medical Technicians and the Emergency Department Nursing Association (EDNA) reflects the trend for increased EMS professionalism.

EMS developments have been encouraged by strong national leadership and substantial funding. When the former Department of Health, Education and Welfare (DHEW) proved reluctant to support EMS, the Department of Transportation (DOT) did so. The reason was hardly obscure: the Department of Transportation was faced with staggering automobile accident statistics, and it acted to improve the motorists' chances of surviving on the road.

> Since 1903, when the 'horseless carriage' toll assumed significance, there have been more than 6,500,000 deaths from accidents in this country, over 1,690,000 involving motor vehicles. In 1965, the accident death toll was approximately 107,000, including 49,000 from motor vehicles...Deaths from traffic injuries have increased annually.[6]

As part of a national highway safety program, the Highway Safety Act of 1966 authorized DOT to fund state agencies for the upgrading of EMS. Those states that did not comply were threatened with the loss of 10 percent of their federal highway construction funds. DOT has awarded over $90 million to the states for improved EMS throughout the country.

DHEW's EMS role expanded in November of 1973 when Congress passed the Emergency Medical Services Systems Act of 1973 (Public Law 93–154), authorizing the department to award up to $185 million for the development of comprehensive regional EMS systems. Local areas receiving such federal seed money were obliged to meet fifteen mandatory criteria that represented a federal blueprint for EMS system development. Among the requirements for EMS systems are trained personnel appropriately distributed, proper communications and transportation systems, and organized emergency facilities. The Emergency Medical Services Amendments of 1976 (Public Law 94–573) continued the federal program, authorizing up to $243 million over a three-year period.

Big government has invested heavily in EMS intervention. Planners in previously disinterested communities have worked with potential EMS administrators in writing applications for funds. At the time of this writing, more than 199 EMS systems are operational. Two hundred more are being called for by DHEW.[7] A ten-year $500 million federal program is anticipated.

System Building: The Job of the Health Administrator

EMS system building is a cooperative effort on the part of many health professionals and community leaders. These leaders most often form an EMS council to set up rational EMS delivery systems and formulate policy. Council members customarily view themselves as partisans serving a well-defined constituency (e.g., the volunteer ambulance squads, the emergency physicians, the hospital staff). The political process is clearly at work here, with all its characteristic bargaining and compromises.

EMS council membership includes the EMS regional administrator, area physicians, nurses, EMTs, hospital administrators, health system agency planners, public safety officials, consumers, and representatives from groups such as the Red Cross, the Heart Association, and Civil Defense. The EMS administrator reports to this council and taps the specialized knowledge of council members.

The size, scope, and setting of the regional program will dictate the type of agency that is to be formed. Nine job titles can be found in regional EMS management organizations: (1) EMS Administrator, (2) Deputy Administrator, (3) Medical Advisor (M.D.), (4) Facilities and Critical Care Specialist, (5) Communications Specialist, (6)

99

Public Information/Education Specialist, (7) Manpower and Training Specialist, (8) Planner/Evaluator, and (9) Field Coordinator.[8]

As is true in other settings, the health administrator as EMS manager gets things done through people—through the EMS council itself and through a staff of specialists reporting to him or her. It is critically important for the administrator to cultivate a working relationship with a prestigious physician who can play a leadership role in system building.

The federal government offers fifteen components as a framework for analyzing the building of an EMS system. These fifteen components are grouped together under broader categories called subsystems in Table 9-1. For each subsystem, selected aspects of the administrator's role will be clarified.

TABLE 9-1

ANATOMY OF AN EMERGENCY MEDICAL SERVICE SYSTEM

I. Training
   Component 1—Manpower
   Component 2—Training
II. Public Education
   Component 3—Public Information and Education
III. Communications
   Component 4—Communications
IV. Field Rescue
   Component 5—Transportation
   Component 6—Public Safety Agencies
   Component 7—Transfer of Patients
V. Facilities
   Component 8—Facilities
   Component 9—Critical Care Units
VI. Management
   Component 10—Consumer Participation
   Component 11—Accessibility to Care
   Component 12—Coordinated Record Keeping
   Component 13—Review and Evaluation
   Component 14—Disaster Linkage
   Component 15—Mutual Aid Agreements

Based on Public Law 93–154, the Emergency Medical Services Systems Act of 1973.

I. Training

Component 1: Manpower: *An adequate number of health professionals, allied health professionals, and other health personnel, including ambulance personnel, with appropriate training and experience.*

Component 2: Training: *The provision for appropriate training (including clinical training) and continuing education programs that (1) are coordinated with other programs in the system's service area which provide similar training and education and (2) emphasize recruitment and necessary training of veterans of the Armed Forces with military training and experience in health care fields, and of appropriate public safety personnel in such areas.*

The training subsystem requires an understanding of new categories of health manpower and the subtleties of the relationships among them.

A minicase involving a 22-year-old graduate student will serve to illustrate potential problems within this subsystem.

E.M. Sledgelug was travelling north on Interstate 95 suffering from sleep deprivation after "cramming for midterms." Sledgelug fell asleep at the wheel, slammed into a pole, and suffered multiple contusions and lacerations with resultant severe bleeding. Responding ambulance paramedics treated Sledgelug appropriately. Among other emergency measures, they applied a MAST suit[9] to elevate the patient's dangerously low blood pressure. (Sledgelug was fortunate in that the paramedics had just completed a training program on the proper use of the MAST suit.)

After stabilizing Sledgelug at the scene, the paramedics transported the patient to a nearby hospital emergency department where two nurses and a physician took over. Unfortunately, these health professionals had not been trained to properly remove a MAST suit. The paramedics were not consulted in the matter, and they were eventually called away to respond to another emergency. Consequently, hospital personnel did an inadequate job of removing the MAST suit. Their negligence (which would never be reported) caused Sledgelug to go into severe shock, rupturing the spleen. Immediate surgery was necessary to save the patient's life.

Sledgelug never completed graduate school and is currently a food service manager at a fried chicken stand.

In this case, Sledgelug was the victim of a common system shortcoming. Training programs for systemwide EMS personnel are not always available, nor are they attended by all who need them. Nurses may refuse to attend classes with EMTs, or physicians will refuse to go to classes with nurses. It is incumbent upon the EMS health administrator (a) to ensure an adequate number of system health personnel, (b) to develop and coordinate appropriate training programs, (c) to create a harmonious atmosphere that maximizes the attainment of system goals, (d) to establish licensure, certification, and recertification criteria, and (e) to improve manpower distribution within the service area.[10]

II. Public Education

Component 3: Public Information and Education: *the EMS system shall provide programs of public education and information for all people in the area, so that they know about the system, how to gain access to it, and how to use it properly.*

Public health and safety education campaigns can help lessen the mortality and morbidity of emergency illness. Yet, such health education is largely neglected and underutilized, possibly because prevention is less exciting than much of EMS. Perhaps administrators and councils are deterred by the intangibility of the long-range rewards of prevention, in contrast to the immediate payoff of other EMS intervention.

The EMS administrator may direct a mass mailing of hundreds of thousands of telephone stickers announcing an emergency access number (such as 911). Or, the EMS agency may work cooperatively with the state or local highway commission to improve highway signing for EMS, telling motorists where to find vital hospital services.

The public is taught first aid, the warning signs of heart attacks, and techniques for the administration of cardiopulmonary resuscitation (CPR). Seattle, Washington, has demonstrated that citizens can become active members of the EMS team by rendering critical first-response CPR to the heart attack victim.[11] Consider the true story of a woman attending a pregame picnic at Memorial Coliseum in Los Angeles:[12]

I saw an older gentleman at a nearby gathering suddenly collapse. A woman (his wife) yelled, "Does anyone here know CPR?" Exactly 24 hours earlier I had completed the Basic Life Support Course. Thus, when I ran to help and found no one else in the crowd capable of administering assistance my training proved invaluable. After sending someone for paramedic help, I then tilted the man's head to assure an open airway; checked his breathing; felt the carotid pulse, and could feel a faint heartbeat. I assisted the unconscious person for approximately 15 minutes, at which time the paramedic group arrived and took over.

101

Like other health administrators, the EMS administrator works in a world of finite resources. If an analysis suggests that funds ought to be expended in the public education area, the administrator may choose to support such a program, even if it is politically unpopular within the EMS system. System personnel may support public education in principle. Yet they may oppose the allocation of limited system resources to public education on the assumption that such allocation diverts monies from ambulance procurement, emergency department upgrading, and other vital EMS activities. The EMS agency will coordinate public education activities with the Heart Association, American Trauma Society, Red Cross, and other civic organizations. Implementing an exciting, effective public education program is rarely easy.

III. Communications

Component 4: Communications: *Provisions for linking the personnel, facilities, and equipment of the system by a central communications system so that requests for emergency health care services will be handled by a communications facility which (1) utilizes emergency telephonic screening, (2) utilizes or will utilize the universal emergency telephone number 911, (3) will have direct communications connections and interconnections with the personnel facilities and equipment of the system and with other appropriate emergency medical services systems, (4) will have the capability to communicate with individuals having auditory handicaps and to communicate in the language of the predominant population groups with limited English-speaking ability in the system's service area, and (5) makes maximum use of communications equipment and systems required under any highway safety program approved under Chapter 4 of Title 23 of the United States Code, and of such equipment and systems acquired under Title I of the Omnibus Crime Control and Safe Streets Act of 1963 (42 U.S.C. 3701 et seq.).*

The EMS administrator wants to grant early citizen access to the EMS system and to ensure communication at the onset of an emergency. The universal emergency telephone number, 911, can provide entry to the regional communications center. If the system is sufficiently developed, a trained EMT working as a dispatcher asks medical questions, gives lifesaving information, and dispatches the most appropriate personnel and equipment.

Here, as in many EMS components, the regionalization concept seems sound. But fundamental questions remain. Why have many different seven-digit emergency phone numbers when a simple 911 alternative is available? Why continue operation of unwieldy sets of municipal dispatch centers, often with poorly trained dispatchers, when one regional center can serve all?

Local providers of service may distrust outsiders. Nevertheless, they can offer persuasive arguments against centralization of EMS. Many have endured frustratingly inefficient service from urban-based dispatchers unacquainted with the geography of outlying areas. Small ambulance companies have lost business when their local dispatcher was supplanted by a regional one. Although communications technology is highly advanced, outlying areas that rely on centralized base stations many miles away complain of weak radio communications that cost lives. A coordinated service requires the regional EMS agency to interface with local EMS providers, police and fire services, and telephone companies. Communications requires specialized knowledge. The administrator works with the communications specialist and service providers in the design and procurement of the communications systems.

IV. Field Rescue

Component 5: Transportation: *This component shall include an adequate number of necessary ground, air, and water vehicles and other transportation facilities properly equipped to meet the transportation and EMS characteristics of the system area. Such vehicles and facilities must meet appropriate standards relating to location, design, performance, and equipment; and the operators and other personnel for such vehicles and facilities must meet appropriate training and experience requirements. (It is expected that "maximum use of vehicles acquired under any highway safety program approved under Chapter 4 of Title 23, United States Code" will be made.)*

Component 6: Public Safety Agencies: *Provisions must be made for effective utilization of appropriate personnel, facilities, and equipment of each public safety agency in the area.*

Component 7: Transfer of Patients: *The EMS system shall provide for transfer of patients to facilities and programs which offer such followup care and rehabilitation as is necessary to effect the maximum recovery of the patient.*

Basic life support systems dispatch EMS ambulance personnel with at least 81 hours of training to the scene in minutes. The EMT can communicate with physicians and nurses via radio and can use an impressive array of medical equipment.

Advanced life support systems include sophisticated ambulances called mobile intensive care units (MICUs), staffed by paramedics with hundreds of hours of training. MICU patients can benefit from space-age technological innovations such as telemetry, which is the radio transmission of a patient's vital signs to a base station. Usually telemetry is used to transmit EKG (heartbeat) signals to a hospital physician, who radios back instructions to the paramedic at the scene. Telemetry is often used to confirm the need for defibrillation (controlled electrical shocks) of patients who are suffering cardiac arrhythmias associated with heart attacks.

These *primary transportation services* are necessary for both basic and advanced life support services. EMS advanced systems must also establish *secondary transportation services* that provide air and ground ambulances for interhospital transfers. These vehicles offer sophisticated services in transporting the stabilized, critically ill patient to a regional critical care center. Secondary transportation services also transfer patients to rehabilitation centers. Fire departments, and, to a lesser extent, police departments, provide prehospital care together with volunteer rescue squads, private ambulance services, and hospital-based services.

Equipment is expensive. An MICU costs over $40,000. Response time in an emergency may be critical. Accordingly, the optimal deployment of transportation equipment is a priority. With the use of computers and other management science techniques, administrators can simulate regional EMS demand and determine the best locations for specific equipment and personnel.

The administrator requests funding from a variety of sources, including the Department of Transportation (DOT) and the Department of Health and Human Services (DHHS), to purchase new equipment, train personnel, and locate these resources within the region. However, the seasoned EMS administrator is aware that regional coordination responsibility does not necessarily mean regional decision-making authority. Local community members will often take exception to regional transportation plans. As with regional communications interventions, local administrators may be wary of loss of control, inadequate coverage of their localities and, of course, the political effects of new regional resource allocations. Volunteer groups occasionally present great problems to the administrator, for they may be highly visible, politically powerful, and locally oriented.

V. Facilities

Component 8: Facilities: *This component shall include an adequate number of easily accessible emergency medical service facilities which are collectively capable of providing service on a continuous (24 hour a day, 7 days a week) basis, which have appropriate standards relating to capacity, location, personnel, and equipment, and which are coordinated with other health care facilities of the system.*

Component 9: Critical Care Units: *This component requires providing access (including appropriate transportation) to specialized critical medical care units.*

These units should be of the number and variety necessary to meet the demands of the service area. If there are no such units in the EMS region, then the system will provide access to units in neighboring areas if this is feasible in terms of time and distance.

DHHS calls on health administrators to develop a regional plan for a coordinated network of emergency facilities. The plan should ensure easy citizen access to the full spectrum of emergency treatment. Administrators must, therefore, take an inventory of the available services offered in area hospital emergency departments and categorize these hospitals on the basis of their ability to deliver emergency care.

There are many types of categorization plans. The American Medical Association (AMA) plan identifies four levels of emergency care facilities based on resources available (both in-house and on-call) at the time of need.[13] The categories are (1) Comprehensive Emergency Service, (2) Major Emergency Service, (3) General Emergency Service, and (4) Basic Emergency Service. A vertical categorization plan is being advanced by DHHS. Under this scheme, hospitals are rated on their ability to deliver services on a disease-specific basis (e.g., trauma, burn).

Categorization of emergency departments is useful to the EMS administrator, to the ambulance dispatcher, and to the general public. EMS administrators need to know about the capabilities of emergency departments in order to make system design decisions. Prehospital personnel need such information in order to transport patients to the most appropriate facility. The public also needs similar facts in order to use the system properly.

Competition among area hospitals and a general wariness of regulation cause many adamantly to oppose the process of categorization. Working through their hospital medical staff committees, physicians may try to block approval of the plan due to fear of losing patients to a more highly rated hospital in the catchment area. Hospital administrators and hospital boards of directors sometimes fear loss of prestige if they fail to be designated as a comprehensive (Type 1) facility.

In contrast, the EMS administrator takes the normative position that categorization of the emergency department does not score overall hospital performance. It would be folly to support a Type 1 emergency department in every hospital in the region, regardless of need.

Using his or her knowledge of categorization, the EMS administrator can identify weak points in the network and upgrade or centralize services as necessary, eliminating redundant services. Many allies will be needed. The administrator customarily works with a leading physician who is committed to gaining acceptance of the program in the medical community. A multidisciplinary team of physicians, nurses, EMTs, and hospital administrators should be actively involved from each of the EMS organizations that will take part in the categorization of facilities.[14]

One administrator invited all hospital administrators, physicians, and nurses in the region to a categorization conference at a local resort. Their task was to help design categorization criteria to be used in the regional plan. The administrator explained that the criteria to be developed would not be used to mandate change, but to aid in the regional planning of a truly comprehensive EMS system. With the assistance of the conferees, the administrator developed a survey instrument that was mailed to all hospital emergency departments for comment. The survey was implemented and the information used for local planning purposes. Emergency departments were categorized, but the information was used by system personnel only. The general public has not been given access to the information.

EMS involves new, untested methods of organization. There is limited evidence thus far to demonstrate that the categorization concept is of value as it is now applied. For the present, the EMS administrator is expected to apply it.

VI. Management

Component 10: Consumer Participation: *The EMS system must make such provisions in its system management that persons residing in the area and having*

104

no professional training or experience may participate in making policy for the system.

Component 11: Accessibility to Care: *The EMS system must provide necessary emergency services to all patients without prior inquiry as to the ability of the patient to pay.*

Component 12: Coordinated Patient Record Keeping: *Each EMS regional system shall provide for a coordinated patient record keeping system which shall cover the patient's treatment from initial entry into the system through his discharge from it, and shall be consistent with patient records used in followup care and rehabilitation.*

Component 13: Review and Evaluation: *Each EMS system must provide the secretary with such information as he may require to conduct periodic, comprehensive, and independent reviews and evaluations of the extent and quality of the emergency health care services provided in the system's service area, and submit to the secretary the results of any review or evaluation which may be conducted by such system of the extent and quality of the emergency health care services provided in the system's service area.*

Component 14: Disaster Linkage: *The EMS system must have a plan to ensure that the system will be capable of providing emergency medical services in the system's service area during mass casualties, natural disasters, or national emergencies.*

Component 15: Mutual Aid Agreements: *Each EMS system must provide for the establishment of appropriate arrangements with EMS systems or similar entities serving neighboring areas for the provision of emergency medical services on a reciprocal basis where access to such services would be more appropriate and effective in terms of services available, time, and distance.*

This subsystem establishes federal requirements for overall system administration. Administrators of EMS programs receiving federal funds need recommendations from consumers, and they must enter into mutual aid agreements with adjacent systems, put together disaster response systems, and carry out systemwide evaluations for DHHS through the use of a uniform patient record keeping system. For the first time in any federal legislation, regional health systems receiving support are ordered to provide emergency medical services to all, regardless of ability to pay.

To maintain continuous operation of the fifteen-element EMS system, the administrator must take an active role in regional financing. This requires knowledge of the sources of grants-in-aid, and the ability to apply for them. Localities are required to raise matching funds in support of the system. There are many ways to finance EMS systems, including funding through tax levies and donations. The use of federal funding obligates service providers to adhere to governmental requirements in areas such as uniform record keeping, accessibility to care, and mutual aid agreements.

Ensuring successful implementation of disaster plans once a major disaster hits can be difficult. The administrator must be available to coordinate services. Physician leadership is indispensable to ensure well-established medical command. The administrator will find it useful to stage mock disaster drills in order to test the readiness of the regional system.

Most organizations that deliver EMS are involved in a broader set of activities. The hospital is committed to delivering a full spectrum of services, only one of which is emergency care. The fire department is committed to putting out and preventing fires. Only during the last several decades have fire departments accepted EMS responsibilities.

These organizations have their own systems of record keeping, and they are not easily persuaded to adopt an externally developed system. Yet gathering uniform data on EMS responses is essential if one is to evaluate its quality. To increase relevance and acceptability, administrators must develop regional management interventions with participation of all who are involved in their use.

Preparing for the Job

EMS health administrators are a varied group. Like their system, they cannot be easily categorized. Many are clinicians: physicians, EMTs, nurses. Some come from backgrounds in public administration. An increasing number enter the field after earning a graduate administrative degree such as the Master of Health Administration (MHA) or the Master of Public Health (MPH). The baccalaureate degree with specialization in EMS administration is also appropriate for certain EMS positions.

EMS administrators can benefit from academic preparation in at least three areas: (1) health care organization, (2) EMS systems development, and (3) administration. Administrators need to comprehend the organization and financing of general health care delivery in order to relate EMS programs to the larger system in which they operate. When dealing with hospital administrators on such issues as categorization of facilities, the EMS administrator must understand hospital decision-making processes, current issues in hospital management, and the relationship of the emergency department to the hospital organization. Innovations in ambulatory care delivery such as health maintenance organizations (HMOs) and the role of the emergency department in ambulatory care delivery are relevant to the development of EMS systems.

Obviously, EMS administrators must master the major concepts and issues relevant to EMS delivery. The EMS system is becoming increasingly complex as substantial funding, technological advances, and innovative methods of delivery increase service capabilities.

The EMS administrator needs the generic skills of the good manager. The EMS administrator needs to understand the theories of management and organizational structure, quantitative methods, computer and information systems, and health institution finances.

The EMS administrator must become a generalist delegator, assigning specific tasks to expert subordinates and consultants.

EMS systems, relying as they do on governmental and foundation funding, require health administrators with proficiency in program planning and proposal writing. Technical writing is important for the administrator who is frequently called upon to develop major reports to EMS constituencies and funding sources. And, of course, administrators must be effective communicators in person-to-person, small groups, and in public speaking situations as well.

Those entering the field with the MHA, MPH, or baccalaureate degree in health administration will bring many of these skills with them. They may be strong in the areas of management and health systems, but may need to develop an in-depth understanding of EMS systems. Health administration graduate and undergraduate programs are beginning to offer courses in EMS systems. Administrators whose competencies are primarily clinical should obtain academic preparation in all of the areas discussed above, with particular emphasis on administration.

Continuing education opportunities exist for the practicing health administrator. The Association of University Programs in Health Administration (AUPHA), in Washington, D.C., has developed a comprehensive educational program for EMS administration. Funded by the Bureau of Health Manpower (BHM) of DHHS, this program is offered by a variety of sponsors at different times of the year. The Center for the Study of Emergency Health Services (CSEHS) at the University of Pennsylvania, and Dunlap and Associates, Inc., in Darien, Connecticut, have both developed educational materials for EMS systems administration under funding by DHHS and DOT, respectively.

The Office of EMS, of DHHS, regularly offers regional and national workshops and conferences on specific aspects of EMS administration for the practicing administrator. Groups such as ACEP and EDNA also offer EMS workshops for their constituencies.

Grounded in general health services administration, perhaps with a specialization in ambulatory care, the recent graduate can take an entry-level or a middle-level job in EMS. Some will specialize in EMS systems throughout their careers. Others will make their mark in EMS and move on to broader health policy and delivery programs. The quality of emergency health services will improve as EMS system leadership develops stronger links with the larger health services administration community.

A Question of Leadership

It has been said that EMS is an infant. Although significant systems developments have occurred over the past decide, little is known about the impact of major EMS systems on regional health indices. Professionals in the field remain optimistic. Workers in the field are experimenting, applying new ideas, looking for fresh perspectives. EMS systems need innovative problem solvers as they continue to develop.

EMS systems development received a mixed report card from the Government Accounting Office (GAO) in its 1976 publication, *Progress, but Problems in Developing Emergency Medical Service Systems*. First, the good news: "EMS systems are probably responsible for the decrease in mortality and disability due to traumatic injury or illness." (GAO's caution reflects the scarcity of verifiable evaluation information.) Now the bad news: "The regional (EMS) concept is being compromised by virtue of the independence and differing priorities of local governments and providers.... Consequently, when Federal funding stops, continuation of regional systems providing service will not be assured in the amounts planned or established with Federal support."

The EMS technology that is already available can be systematized to save lives and reduce illness. Will system building cease for lack of local initiative? The answer depends on the present and the future caliber of the EMS administrator.

NOTES

[1]The 1972 amendments to the Social Security Act provide for the creation of Professional Standards Review Organizations (PSROs) designed to involve local practicing physicians in the ongoing review and evaluation of health care services covered under the Medicare, Medicaid, and Maternal and Child Health Programs.

[2]Gerald A. Doesken, Jack Frye, and Bernall Green, *Economics of Rural Ambulance Service in the Great Plains*. Washington, D.C.: U.S. Department of Agriculture, Economic Development Division, Economic Research Service Pub. No. 308, 1975.

[3]Robert E. Motley, Department of Transportation, National Highway Traffic Safety Administration, Washington, D.C. Private interview, August 1976.

[4]Cambridge Research Institute, *Trends Affecting the U.S. Health Care System*. U.S. Department of Health, Education and Welfare, HRA 76-14503, 1975, p. 262. Much of this increase is caused by ambulatory overload. In many communities, the hospital emergency department has replaced the family physician as the source of primary health care services. Sixty percent of all emergency department visits may be non-emergency walk-ins with no other source of care.

[5]Committee on Public Policy of American College of Emergency Physicians, "Emergency Medical Services: Problems, Programs and Policies." East Lansing, Michigan: American College of Emergency Physicians, 1977.

[6]National Academy of Sciences/National Research Council, *Accidental Death and Disability: The Neglected Disease of Modern Society.* Washington, D.C., 1966. p. 8.

[7]"It's an Emergency." *Newsweek,* November 21, 1977. p. 108.

[8]James O. Page, J.D., "EMS Manpower and Training." *Educational Program for EMS Systems Administration and Planning.* Washington, D.C.: AUPHA, 1977. pp. 33–37.

[9]MAST stands for Medical Anti-Shock Trousers.

[10]Page, *op. cit.* (note 8).

[11]"Seattle Emergency Plan Is Saving Heart Victims," *New York Times,* January 21, 1975, p. 59.

[12]*EMS Action.* January 1978. ACT Foundation, New Jersey.

[13]American Medical Association, *Categorization of Emergency Capabilities.* Chicago: American Medical Association, 1971.

[14]D.R. Boyd, "Categorization of Emergency Medical Capabilities of Hospitals." Hyattsville, Maryland,: HEW, Division of EMS, 1975.

[15]*Progress, but Problems in Developing Emergency Medical Service Systems.* Washington, D.C.: Government Accounting Office, 1976.

REFERENCES

American Academy of Orthopedic Surgeons, Committee on Injuries. *Emergency Care and Transportation of the Sick and Injured.* Chicago: American Academy of Orthopedic Surgeons, 1971.

Andrews, Robert B. *Methodologies for the Evaluation and Improvement of Emergency Medical Services Systems.* U.S. Department of Transportation, National Highway Traffic Safety Administration. DOT HS-801 848. Washington, D.C.: U.S. Government Printing Office, 1975.

Doeksen, Gerald A., and Jack Frye. *Economics of Rural Ambulance Service in the Great Plains.* U.S. Department of Agriculture, Economic Development Division, Economic Research Service. U.S. Government Printing Office, 1975.

"Emergency Medical Services." *Hospitals, Journal of the American Hospital Association* 47, 10 (1973).

Gibson, Geoffrey. "Regionalization and Emergency Medical Services: The Dance of the Lemmings." *Regionalization and Health Policy,* Eli Ginzburg, ed., Washington, D.C.: Department of Health, Education and Welfare, 1978.

Jenkins, Astor L. *Emergency Department Organization and Management.* St. Louis: The C.V. Mosby Company, 1975.

Motley, Robert E., Department of Transportation, National Highway Traffic Safety Administration, Washington, D.C. Private interview, August 1976.

Noble, John H., *et al. Emergency Medical Services: Behavioral and Planning Perspectives.* New York: Behavioral Publications, 1973.

Page, James O. *Emergency Medical Services for Fire Departments* (2d ed.) NFPA Publication No. FSP–45. Boston: The National Fire Protection Association, 1978.

Rockwood, Charles A., Jr., *et al.* "History of Emergency Medical Services in the United States." *Journal of Trauma* 4 (April 1976):pp. 229–308.

U.S. Congress. *Emergency Medical Services Systems Act of 1973.* P.L. 93–154, 42 U.S.C. §201 *et seq.* (1976).

U.S. Department of Health, Education and Welfare. *Accidental Death and Disability: The Neglected Disease of Modern Society.* Emergency Health Series A-13, Public Health Service Publication No. 1071-A-13, Washington, D.C.: U.S. Government Printing Office, 1966.

U.S. Department of Health, Education and Welfare. *Emergency Medical Services System Program Guidelines.* Publication No. (JSC) 75–2013. Washington, D.C.: U.S. Government Printing Office, 1975.

Yolles, Tamarath K. "Emergency Medical Service Systems: A Concept Whose Time Has Come." *Journal of Emergency Nursing* 1 (July–August 1975): pp. 31-36.

10   As Health Policy Analyst

Patricia Bauman, M.P.H.

Public officials, whether elected or appointed, have to be fast learners, but they are never omniscient. They cannot be expected personally to stay on top of everything, even in selected fields. Consequently, they need conscientious staff advisors who do stay abreast of events. This is important, particularly in the area of health care with its costly technology, its contending institutions and personnel, its labyrinthine funding, its suboptimal service distribution, and its highly political nature. Health policy analysts gather and analyze information, and counsel their superiors. Staff analysts may assiduously cultivate anonymity, but insiders know the magnitude of their influence on the formulation and implementation of health policies.

Like her colleagues, Patricia Bauman has worked as a health administrator in more than one setting. Here she describes how satisfactions outweigh frustrations for the health policy analyst who expects a long-term social payoff in the form of increasingly available and effective health care. (L.E.B.)

Introduction

For two years, it was my privilege to serve on the staff of the U.S. Senate Committee on Human Resources for its Ranking Minority Member, Senator Jacob K. Javits of New York. I was assigned to its Subcommittee on Health and Scientific Affairs. At the time this chapter was written, thirty professionals worked on the Subcommittee's business, either as staff to the Committee itself allocated to a particular Senator, or as Senators' personal staff assigned by them to health care and other issues. Three of the thirty had taken graduate degrees in health administration, and of four physicians, two held degrees in public health as well. Those without formal academic preparation in the health field included nine lawyers, a political scientist, a few people with previous staff experience within the Department of Health, Education and Welfare (HEW) [now the Department of Health and Human Services (HHS)], and a group who had learned about health policy analysis on the job. The staff configurations are flexible and vary at different times and among different congressional committees or executive departments. However, staff who are engaged in common tasks in a particular setting generally have diverse educational preparation and work experience.

Patricia Bauman, M.P.H., is a consultant for the National Institute of Environmental Health Sciences (N.I.H.).

Patricia Bauman was a Professional Staff Member of the U.S. Senate Committee on Human Resources when this chapter was written. The views and opinions expressed are her own and do not reflect those of the Committee or its Ranking Minority Member at that time, Senator Jacob K. Javits, on whose staff for the Committee she served.

The author is grateful to J. David Banta and Bess Dana for their helpful criticism of the manuscript.

Every level of government has broadened its involvement in health care activities, including health policy problems, the solutions to which health administrators can contribute. Nevertheless, the government job market for health policy analysts who will generate policy options and develop legislation is small in comparison to the large numbers of graduates from proliferating health policy programs under the auspices of schools of law, social work, public health, business administration, public administration, urban planning, and other interdisciplinary programs. Since small working groups and task forces seem to work well for governmental policy decision making, they are preferred to offices with large numbers of analysts.

Thus, many professions compete for the relatively few health policy jobs available in the federal government: as staff to congressional committees; as personal staff assigned to health matters; as staff to the Secretary of Health, Education and Welfare; as staff to other officials of HEW, such as the Assistant Secretary for Health and the Deputy Assistant Secretary for Planning and Evaluation; as health policy staff to the Office of Management and Budget (OMB); and as staff to the White House.[1] Health administrators in such jobs will find that their specialized training is useful. But they will be likely also to find that health policy analysts in government are more akin to each other than to other health administrators, at least while they hold staff jobs.

Important differences exist in the nature of the work and in substance and style between local and federal government. Within Congress, there are differences between House and Senate, differences among the various committees, differences between personal and committee staff, differences between majority or minority party, and so on. Comparable variations are found within and among executive departments as well. I shall allude to some of these, but my principal focus will be on the generic aspects of the staff role of health policy analysts in government.

First, and most important is the truism that policy analysis in all settings is generated within a political context; that is, there is no such thing as a value-free policy environment that spawns zero-based analysis. As a corollary, the effective analyst recognizes and operates within the political constraints of his or her particular world.[2] The contented analyst respects the legitimacy of the political process of bargaining, compromise, negotiation, and, as a rule, incremental adjustments that happen within and between executive and legislative branches of government, and between government and the outside world. The second generic similarity lies in the aggregate of satisfactions and frustrations health policy analysts are likely to experience, whatever their place in the political structure. Finally, regardless of the original field in which the analyst was grounded, he or she accumulates a group of new skills.

Life on the Hill

During the relative lull of the summer congressional recess, Senator Javits's health staff pondered potential legislation to address problems of urban health care organization and delivery to accompany his national health insurance bill for mothers and children. We had sifted through more than one hundred letters of criticism and suggestions that the Senator had requested from a spectrum of experts and parties interested in this bill. We had reviewed the public hearings on the companion measure in the House of Representatives. We had digested the critique of the bill that had been prepared at our request by the Congressional Research Service, an analytic resource of the Congress. Accordingly, we now felt ready to meet with Legislative Counsel and staff representing the principal sponsor in the House in order to redraft the bill to reflect new policy changes. Afterwards, we planned to make an inventory of these changes in detail, with careful justification, for the Senator's use as he made the final judgments on each of our specific recommendations. Later this memorandum would serve as the basis for the Senator's floor statement accompanying the new bill, for letters to constituents seeking his views on national health insurance, and for the "Dear Colleague" letter that would seek cosponsorship.

The Senator is not a member of the Committee on Finance, which has principal jurisdiction over national health insurance (NHI) in the Senate. Nevertheless, he has been immersed in health issues for more than a decade, and he has strong views about relevant social policy assumptions and choices for NHI. We knew that NHI initiatives were being planned by the Carter administration, so we concluded that the NHI issue would be more active than it had been under Nixon or Ford. The Senator agreed that he should continue to contribute fruitfully to the national discussion. None of us, including and probably especially the Senator, was dismayed by the certain knowledge that his bill, as written, would never become the law of the land. Nevertheless, it was gratifying to realize that the Senator's goals and objectives might well be represented in the final, compromise outcome.

As we were modifying "Kiddycare," as we irreverently but affectionately termed it, we got the Senator's blessing to transfer part of the bill, providing support for group practices, and use it in another bill. This new broadly focused bill would help reorganize health care delivery, particularly in cities, with their problems of poorly distributed resources, concomitant waste, and barriers to access.

We had met informally with HEW staffers responsible for the Community Health Centers program to determine how their ideas for tackling urban health problems coincided with our own, and to ascertain, with their anonymous consent, which of their ideas we might incorporate into a draft bill. I had consulted with my former colleagues in the Department of Community Medicine at the Mount Sinai School of Medicine to learn firsthand about current progress and problems in health services planning and delivery in East Harlem, and I had come away with new information about programs that could serve as adaptable models for legislation. We had met with officials of public and voluntary hospitals to learn about their problems. We were awaiting legislative recommendations and draft language that we had requested from a consultant to the American Hospital Association concerning how the government might assist hospitals in meeting one-time costs of achieving long-term cost savings through closing beds, merging and regionalizing services, and the like. In the meantime, we were improving the original group practice part of the bill with the help of an expert in the Health Maintenance Organization (HMO) program at HEW. The Senator's well-known interest in sponsoring a bill to alleviate urban health problems continued to attract ideas and offers of help and criticism from new contacts.

Should the Senator's urban health proposal focus on improving access to services, especially for groups like the working poor? Should it concentrate on health planning in general and resource development in particular? Should it assist hard-pressed facilities like municipal hospitals or outpatient departments? Or, should it pick and choose, with no particular unifying theme, among the range of health policy problems that require resolution or, at least, discussion?

Normally we would not have had time to dwell excessively on such conceptual questions. However, it was August. Pressures upon staff had lessened. There were no committee meetings requiring staff preparation, no expiring legislative authorities demanding analysis and possible amendment, and no other Senator's bills or amendments on which to comment. There were fewer speeches to draft, and fewer interest groups and other constituents to meet. We luxuriated in this time for contemplation of fundamental questions, although I suspect we looked forward to the customary frantic pace.

Variety and lack of a predictable agenda typify the staffer's life as I experienced it. Seeking and processing information, communicating with numerous people on numerous subjects, and assisting decision makers fill the days of the staff person in the policy-making arenas of government. Standing anonymously behind the Congress, behind a Senator or Representative, behind the President, behind the Secretary and other officials, are the analytic staff who work on the executive and legislative proposals that are subject always to the test of the political process. No elected or appointed official could make decisions without the help of such staff. As every staffer (and every assistant administrator) knows, the elected or appointed officials ultimately take responsibility for decisions in a politically defined world.

The Political Context of Health Policy Analysis

Since the policy process consists of defining goals and setting forth and comparing ways of achieving them,[3] policy analysis deals with both means and ends.[4] Environmental constraints of the real world affect both how problems are characterized and what strategies may be selected. These include such basic facts of institutional life as mission, tradition, available resources (including expertise, personnel, money), existing or possible programs within an organization's jurisdiction, relationships with and expectations held by outside constituencies, and political alliances—all of which focus or limit an organization's choices. For all practical purposes, the analyst will find that much of his environment is in fact already set in place. A policy world in which analysts start from scratch on purely rational grounds—assuming that rationality is ever pure—is a technologist's fantasy and a democrat's nightmare.[5] The health staffer who wants to reduce frustration will recognize that analysis is but one ingredient of decision making, its relative importance determined by the issue at hand. The staffer's task may well be to combine policy research, raw data, and technical information with other kinds of advice such as political intelligence. Even so, his recommendations may be overridden for a wide variety of reasons that he may never discover.[6]

The most important aspect of one's political environment is what might be called, for want of a better term, its moral or ethical climate. For example, I would not have applied for a job with Senator Javits if there had been a poor ideological fit, nor would I have been hired. Had I slipped into the staff anyway, I would have performed badly on the job. The reverse was true, so as I expected, I was proud and happy to be on his staff. It is a serious mistake, so I believe, ever to work for a person or an agency whose world view is discordant with one's own—although I do not imply that a robot-like agreement on all matters at all times is necessary, or even desirable. People and their surroundings change, so that an analyst may find his earlier sense of comfort challenged. In that event a rigorous re-evaluation is needed, followed perhaps by a resignation.[7]

During my job interviews I was not asked about my political affiliation, but I was asked—and I in turn inquired—about basic health and social policy predilections, values, and inclinations. The preselection process, wherein policy staff tend to share basic approaches to problems both with each other and with their bosses, is similarly a feature in cabinet departments and agencies in the executive branch.[8] This congruence is so pervasive and so necessary because policy and politics are closely linked. Thus, staff advice perceived as useful is advice harmonious with the political needs and orientation of the decision maker who requested it.

Sometimes appreciation of political realities or the particular situation of one's employer overrides an impressively thoughtful exchange of information and analysis.[9] When I first came to work in the Senate, our committee's major effort centered around drafting and redrafting the bill that finally became the "Health Professions Educational Assistance Act of 1976" (Public Law 94–484). I was struck by the intellectual quality of the staff markup sessions, at which most differences among members of the committee are ironed out and then cleared and approved by the legislators before they themselves meet as a group. These sessions often seemed like sophisticated graduate seminars. Staff were open-minded, versed in many substantive issues, and familiar with the professional literature. At one long and contentious meeting, however, a senior staff member for the Health Subcommittee Chairman (Senator Edward M. Kennedy), a veteran of a decade on the Hill, revealingly noted, "This conversation typifies the whole process. We can be rational on substantive issues. But when we're being run down the gangplank politically, we have to behave like raving maniacs, and substance goes out the window."

We may allow for hyperbole born of fatigue and pressure, but clearly he was alluding to a truth that not everyone is temperamentally suited to handle: when assertiveness and sweet reason fail, one must occasionally be prepared to engage in combat. As a rule, though, legislative staff resemble their bosses in recognizing the need to get along with colleagues over the long haul and minimize conflict. Spending too much of one's energy and ego on a single issue, no matter what the rights or the wrongs, exhausts supplies of effort and credibility for the next battle.

Such is the climate for compromise. Political realities determine the bread-and-butter substance of the health policy analyst's work, first by defining the scope and focus of the government in which he works. For the work of Congress is done in committees, each of which has jurisdiction over executive branch departments, agencies, and programs that are authorized—and increasingly required to be reauthorized—by legislation. The jurisdictional turfs of the committees have grown by accretion, tradition, internal politicking, and empire-building. The same comment applies to the executive branch. Occasionally, collective wisdom, experience, and the emergence of pressing social problems like environment or energy in new and salient forms lead to governmental reorganizations.[10] In 1977 this happened in the Senate in the restructuring of congressional committees. Nevertheless, the fragmentation, gaps, and duplications deplored by efficiency experts seem inevitable in a very complex world where large problems have to be divided into reasonably manageable pieces.[11]

In Congress, expiring legislative authorities, hearings and other oversight activities, and the budget process all demand attention before new legislation is considered.[12] Usually congressional committees limit serious review of bills to those sponsored by their own members, and the chairman thus exerts considerable power by setting committee schedules and agenda. In deference to the committee structure, my colleagues and I focused on programs already or likely to be subject to the Public Health Service Act when we considered new legislation, since the Committee on Human Resources has jurisdiction over it.

We did not begin with the global question of how to help people in cities achieve a healthier life. Thus we excluded environmental matters (under Senate jurisdiction of the Committee on Public Works and Environment), nutrition (under the Committee on Agriculture and Nutrition), and welfare reform (under the Committee on Finance), —to cite a few of several areas of potential consideration. Nor did we place major emphasis on financing programs like Medicare and Medicaid to alter the health system, since these are in the domain of the Committee on Finance.[13] Our question instead became, What is the very best we can do with what we have? We also asked, Can we expand our borders just a bit by using financing for leverage? I did not feel intellectually dishonest or lazy in accepting these limits: this is life in the world of policymaking.

The executive branch has similar constraints, as I discovered in my first job in New York City's Health Services Administration. My task there was to prepare a critique of a proposed sickle-cell anemia screening program that was to be included in an existing lead poisoning control program. I suggested instead the approach of voluntary screening and counseling for at-risk groups seeking marriage licenses. The given, which was certainly not open to serious challenge by a staffer, was that something had to be done about sickle-cell anemia. The community wanted a program; the Mayor wanted a program; the agency intended to create one; and I tried to come up with one that was at least plausible, based on my best analytic efforts and common sense. An executive department also inherits many existing programs that are hard to change or replace.

The style or personality of the setting defines much of the environment of the health policy analyst. Fenno[14] and Price[15] cogently describe these differences among congressional committees. Polsby[16] characterizes basic differences in the standard operating procedures[17] of the House and Senate. Scholars and observers note abiding characteristics of executive departments and agencies.[18] The types of senators and representatives who gravitate towards particular committees tend to be fairly consis-

115

tent over time. A strong chairman can make a difference, but committees, like executive agencies, tend to have lives of their own. The Committee on Human Resources, for instance, is much more liberal, activist, and oriented to Big Government than is the Committee of Finance, which is known for its conservatism. This difference in committee styles may be more significant than political party to legislative outcome. It is not surprising that staff, too, should share these differences. There is a general like-mindedness among colleagues on a particular committee staff, and in their collaboration with staff from other committees there is sometimes competition, and sometimes the need to make a mental adjustment to other world views.

Cozy triumvirates, iron triangles, and similar terms that describe long-standing relationships among congressional committees, agency personnel, and relevant interest groups reinforce the personality of the policy environment for the analyst. The process by which career civil service professionals consult informally with legislative staff to share expertise and criticism and actually to draft bills together is a very common one and is perceived to be beneficial all around. The Nixon administration tried unsuccessfully to stop this practice. It had correctly noted that the collaborative practice gives bureaucrats direct access to Congress, albeit anonymously, while they bypass the upper echelons of politically appointed policymakers.

Interest groups, too, provide valuable information, technical expertise, data, and first-hand experience about programs and problems to executive agencies and especially to Congress, which has fewer resources for data collection and analysis. A health staffer in both branches can and does tap many sources for ideas and information. There are experts in universities and foundations, or lobbyists for large organizations like the Association of American Medical Colleges or the American Hospital Association. There are spokesmen for single-focus groups like the American Society for Medical Technologists or the Group Health Association of America. These representatives of the outside world, who comprise the third leg of the triangle, share a common environment with the people who pass the laws and the people who implement the programs that affect them. Interest group participation helps to gain support and defuse opposition, and interest group members experienced in government processes may function as bridges between people in the two branches of government who are not in direct contact with each other or who may not know of each other's mutual interest. The analyst quickly gets to know the other people who inhabit the same policy world, wherever they are.

The Political Context: Contrasts in Tasks and Attitudes in the Executive and Legislative Branches

Health policymaking is a political function, and thus is located in a political structure. However, the analytic staff in the executive branch is often more remote from an explicit scrutiny of the political implications of its analytic work than is the case for congressional staff. The people who look at policy alternatives from the vantage of political realism in the executive are generally not the same people who first generated these options. A third kind of staff function entails developing legislative proposals for submission to Congress and serving as liaison with congressional staff. One health policy analyst in the executive branch, describing how his environment affected his ability to make a difference, referred to himself as a technician rather than a politician (who bravely takes independent initiative).[20]

The congressional staff are given quite a different charge. An elected Senator or Representative must always think about getting re-elected at some point, no matter how safe the seat.[21] As a result, his staff tend to think automatically about who wins and who loses in any policy decision. The professional staff also hear from concerned constituents who unambiguously express their views. Therefore, the test of political feasibility is seen immediately and is perceived as much more essential by analysts in Congress than by their counterparts in the executive branch.[22] Staff generally include germane interest group analysis[23] (which can spell the difference between an idea's

116

success and its failure) in briefing memos for their bosses.[24] This immediate feedback means that, compared to executive branch staff, congressional staff tend to be occupied more with process than substance. Happily, both deserve attention in our democratic system of government. Certainly, most major efforts to address complex social problems are generated in the executive branch, and Congress then reacts to them, often creatively.

Despite the differences, all health policy analysts in government live in the same political world as their bosses, and must live with some of the same problems. Decision makers must use judgment and common sense as they act in the face of uncertainty, time pressure, and conflicting interests. So do staff who produce the option papers, briefing memoranda, testimony, amendments, and the like. Staff, therefore, must make clear to their bosses the difference between fact and their own judgment, between relative certainty and hunch.

Staff cope with these pressures by seeking information, opinion, advice, and analysis from a variety of sources: hence the cooperation among groups in the triumvirates rather than an adversary relationship between government and the outside world. This coziness has been criticized on the grounds that some voices are heard more distinctly than others,[25] but several factors keep a health staffer honest.

First, getting advice is not synonymous with taking it. For example, when we consulted with the American Hospital Association staff about ways to encourage regionalization of tertiary care, we all knew in advance that we might not agree. We all realized that the Senator might choose to use all or part or none of their recommendations. Nor would the Senator necessarily support the Association's position on other matters. No sophisticated interest group expects uncritical acceptance, and those that use the hard sell are not respected.

The second factor keeping the staffer honest, especially the legislative staffer, is the need to listen and to be available to constituents, to be both courteous and openminded. In particular, it is common practice to search out the experience of people from a member's home state or district. Therefore, Senator Javits's staff talked to New York City hospital administrators when analyzing problems of urban hospitals nationwide. Just as a member's personal staff respond to problems of individual constituents, so do committee staff respond to its constituency groups, local and national.

The final factor contributing to the staffer's honesty, is his or her knowledge that the proverbial buck stops with the member of Congress. Likewise in the executive branch the cabinet official is responsible to the President for decisions made and policies adopted, and the President is ultimately accountable. Recent history teaches us afresh that these systems can break down, but they appear remarkably resilient. In an interesting column in *The Washington Post*, Stanley Karnow concludes that the multifaceted pulling and tugging of the political process prevents staff excesses. Karnow notes that "...the fragmentation of the legislature has made the congressional staff increasingly influential. For, senators and representatives are functioning more independently than they ever have, and like autonomous barons, they rely heavily on their staffs."[26] He may or may not be correct in noting that congressional staff are often more powerful than their counterparts in the administration, but I have observed that staff in both branches of government have respect for the particular responsibility and accountability that go with making decisions.

Certainly Senator Javits poses the toughest questions to his staff. The Senator judges quickly whether a recommendation is right for him or not, and why. He very freely rejects advice and ideas, while proposing others he wishes to pursue. The Senator trusts his staff, although he watches them closely.

Policy activists have to live in harmony because they share a small world in which they frequently cross the semipermeable membrane between private and public sectors,[27] or between executive government and Congress, moving in and out of universities, research institutes, medical schools, interest groups, and so on. The community of health policy analysts is fluid yet filled with familiar faces. During the Nixon and

Ford administrations there was an informal government in exile of liberal Democrats on the Hill and Academe, many of whom have now returned as political lawyer health analysts in the Department of Health, Education and Welfare under the Carter administration. Civil service staff may be detailed to the White House or other policymaking offices, or may serve as congressional fellows. Congressional staff, having caught Potomac Fever or having become interested in pursuing a particular subject in depth, may seek the opportunity for greater concentration afforded by work in a line agency. Or they may work for an interest group. Naturally, there is some turnover and new blood. Moreover, as people shift institutional auspices, they expand their knowledge and appreciation of different interests and points of view. This movement of health policy analysts in and out of government encourages and rewards, by means of seniority and key positions, those who are incrementalists or very patient bargainers.

The Political Context: Its Impact on Satisfactions and Frustrations

If one can abide the frustrations, then the rewards of health policy work in government are enormous. Frustration tolerance is probably a matter of personality type; one has to be able to recognize that one cannot change the world, except in very small ways. The health policy analyst must know that some of his vigorous and most intelligent efforts will come to naught, lost in the political maze. With so many countervailing pressures, the outcome of the democratic process often reflects everyone's relative impotence. Critics decry our lack of the comprehensive national health policy that they argue is essential if we are to attack public health problems, which demand planned, rather than incremental, actions. Most analysts, though, prefer to slog along step by step (while privately holding some long-range personal ideals) rather than to try to impose their notions of the public good on the rest of the world, or to find themselves imposed upon with someone else's notion of it. At the same time, I think we all feel a tension between pragmatism and idealism that can be painful at times. And, for better or worse, there is little room for radicals in this setting.

The result of a realistic self-perception of one's own limits and those of the political process need not be cynicism or amorality. On the contrary, part of the satisfaction of the job derives from expressing and giving substance to one's personal values. At the same time, fundamental respect for the messiness of democracy, for the legitimacy of the other person's interests, is essential for personal and professional happiness. The difficult task is to learn to lose gracefully while deciding where to take a stand and try to win. These observations hold whether one is putting together or advocating an executive proposal or negotiating on behalf of and under the supervision of a member of Congress. Graceful defeat is a matter of style and practice; but actually losing on an issue about which one has strongly held beliefs is never a pleasant experience.

There is also the heady feeling that comes from seeing one's ideas embodied in a statute or in an executive policy or in an actual program. It *is* possible to make a difference, even if it is miniscule. However, a staffer in Congress, for instance, errs in trying to take credit for legislative achievements that in fact belong to the legislator himself.

It is sobering to keep in mind one's personal and organizational limitations when one is being courted and flattered. I have never encountered an instance among my health analyst colleagues of influence peddling, in the newspaper exposé sense of the term. But health analysts find themselves sought after and deferred to by high government officials, by scholars, and by professionals, whom health analysts may have held in awe from afar. The health staffer who places a telephone call on behalf of Senator So-and-So should recognize that the prompt response is to him only as the Senator's agent. A healthy dose of humility is in order, even while the staffer enjoys being the legislator's eyes and ears for the outside world. This situation gives the legitimate opportunity to establish a personal reputation based on one's professional skills and integrity.

I judge that most health policy analysts are self-starting activists, with at least a touch of the entrepreneur. There is room for entrepreneurship in the executive branch, where there is always a search for ideas to solve problems related to health issues. Regardless of which political party is in the White House, if government wants to control costs, to limit and consolidate its activities, and to ration rather than expand resources, it needs health policy analysts. The field is a growth industry in subject area, although few people are hired to do the job.

Each member assigns staff people to different functional areas, and the size of his or her staff depends on the district represented, seniority, and rank on committees. The health policy analyst learns to be assertive lest he or she lose out in the competition among the staff for the boss's attention. The health staffer in Congress must never forget that health policy is but one of many legitimate areas of interest to his or her employer, and possibly not preeminent at that.

Life as a health policy analyst is not for everyone, certainly not for purists who think that rational solutions ought to prevail over dirty politics. It is not a life for those who feel uneasy about making judgments under terrible time constraints with limited and uncertain information, nor is it a life for those who are steeped in a particular academic discipline and who feel uncomfortable working with a motley, diverse group of colleagues and constituents. And the life of the health policy analyst in Congress in particular is not for those who only enjoy thinking globally and who insist on drawing up blueprints to create major and rapid change. Nevertheless, to participate in the political process, however incremental and intangible the results, is usually a profoundly rewarding intellectual and emotional experience for the health policy analyst.

Eventually many analysts reach a point when the excitement of the process may become routine. The constant contact with people, even important ones, no longer seems quite so glamorous. It may even seem less significant to have had some role in a policy outcome. At such a time the frantic pace and the frustrations of not being able to delve into issues, of reacting to crises, and of losing one's substantive skills can begin to wear the health staffer down. It then comes home to the health policy analyst that the work is generally not a lifetime vocation. But to have gained an understanding of the political process in all its complexity casts new light on one's past professional contributions in health administration.

Skills and Training

The particular substantive knowledge and skills of the health administrator contribute most to health policy analysis in government when they are fused with personality attributes of flexibility, open-mindedness, and strength of ego. Skills and knowledge alone do not suffice. Like their colleagues from the fields of law, medicine, economics, and public administration, health administrators must be able to seek out, sift, synthesize, and assess critically a wide range of information—technical, scholarly, and political—and apply the fruits of these labors to a policy problem. In assembling the best possible intelligence, in analyzing its quality and relevance, and in adding political realities to the calculus of judgment, policy analysts must be discerning consumers first and foremost.

Logical thinking, which is—or ought to be—at the core of professional training, is thus a *sine qua non*. Rigorous training in application of the scientific method will stand the health policy analyst in good stead. For the health administrator, a particularly valuable element of the academic curriculum, one with wide and subtle applicability, is epidemiology. Mastery of this discipline, with its emphasis on definition and measurement, on the importance of how questions and hypotheses are formulated, on methodology, on identifying the underlying assumptions and the limitations of the data at hand, on reformulating and retesting hypotheses in the light of new knowledge, enriches the quality of the health analyst's work.[28] When facing a blizzard of studies and reports, it is often tempting to read the findings and skip the questions and methods. When one plans actually to use something, though, it is worth trying to apply epidemiologic discipline and read as critically and carefully as possible.

Epidemiology deals with the distribution of health and illness in population groups, and so must health policy. Concepts of probability, of relative risk, of validity all enter into the making of sound judgments. Again, it must be stressed that policy is not made solely or even primarily on technical or even logical grounds. For example, it would not be good policy, nor would it be politically feasible, simplistically to allocate dollars for categorical disease research proportional to disease-specific mortality rates without a consideration of factors like state of research progress in a field, public concern and salience, or costs. Anecdote and the individual case history certainly affect policy, but so does the type of analysis in which the epidemiologist's question is asked "How does that incident compare with others?"

Since analysts have to assess the reasonableness of the intelligence they consume, a good working knowledge of the health care field—how it is organized and financed, what its resources are, how its social systems operate—is very helpful. This knowledge comes from the general curriculum of health administration and first-hand experience practicing in the field. So health administrators bring a special perspective to the deliberations they share with colleagues from other fields. Since those who inhabit the policy world speak in many tongues, it is imperative that they be comfortable with the vocabulary and fundamentals of economics, sociology, and political science. It is not necessary to be a lawyer to write a bill or amendment, since the analyst can work with the agency or the congressional counsel who will translate policy ideas into legislative language. Still, it is essential to be able to read and understand legislation and administrative regulations.

Another important skill for the analyst—one that is rarely taught in professional schools—is the ability to write quickly and reasonably well. Speeches, statements, memoranda, reports, and letters are the principal modes of communication in health policy work, so that the analyst has to command a simple, clear expository prose style. Indeed, a job candidate should be prepared to produce samples of his or her writing. Good writing may seem a trivial or self-evident, or even old-fashioned and obsolete, attribute, but government runs on the printed word. Many an argument has triumphed, many a decision maker has been persuaded, and many a decisive point has been won by skillful use of ordinary English that rises above thickets of jargon and obfuscation. The related skill of speed-reading saves much time. In its absence, selective skimming becomes an intuitive art.

The Health Administrator in the Job Market

Perhaps there is no such animal as a policy analyst.[29] Certainly those who comprise the field of health administration can claim no exclusive analytic competence. People who have training in health administration can and do have important public policy positions, but the range of expertise required to address problems at hand is so broad, and personality attributes so pre-eminent over formal training, that policy analysts will always represent many professions and disciplines. Ellwood notes that an economic orientation is typical of the executive branch, while lawyers and physicians predominate in the Congress.[30] Congressional style is inductive, deriving general principles from specific cases—precisely the way physicians and lawyers are trained to think. Sometimes staff members cluster according to their education. When I was serving in the New York City Health Services Administration, for example, the majority of health policy positions were held by business school graduates, who were in fashion at that time and in that place.

Health administrators have earned respect and continue to gain stature in government health policy making. However, a lawyer or a physician will still find it easier to get a foot in the door and find a job. The status gap may be shrinking, but it still exists. Once accepted, the analyst's individual merit counts for far more than academic credentials. Getting hired, in fact, is often just a matter of luck, personal connections, or sheer persistence in getting the job interview when a place opens up. There are enough good people available to preclude cronyism. I cannot think of anyone who holds a job in health policy as a result of political favoritism, but there are many who got their jobs through an Old Boy Network among professionals.

There are more opportunities for researchers in health policy than for staff to government policymakers. These, too, represent a variety of professions and academic disciplines. Despite an uncertain climate in which research must constantly justify its germaneness to policy,[31] health policy research and its recommendations do in fact enter into decision making. The major governmental loci for such research are the line agencies of the Public Health Service, the Social Security Administration, the National Center for Health Services Research, and the National Institutes of Health. This list excludes other Departments such as Defense, the Veterans' Administration, Environmental Protection Agency, Department of Labor, and others that deal with health matters directly or indirectly. Government also seeks health policy research and advice from universities and medical schools, and from for-profit consulting firms and non-profit research institutes.

A consideration of the content, skills, and satisfactions of policy research would take us far beyond the scope of this discussion, but the lines between research and advice are often blurry in health issues. Therefore, it is not uncommon for researchers to take sabbaticals from the civil service or Academe into the messy world of real politics. Nor is it unheard of for policy activists in government to enter or return to academic or government agency research. People who build these kinds of career bridges are in a good position to know what kinds of researchable questions may be useful to decision makers and how to design and present their work accordingly. Conversely, if they enter government policymaking with previous research experience, they are likely to be good critics of the information they used to gather. Such people are not wedded to their disciplines as a rule, and they like to see their research—or their policy analyses—applied to problems in the political arena.

The Health Administrator's Contribution to Government Policy Analysis

As the committee staff meetings ranged about the directions of medical education and the nature of government's support of health personnel training, I found myself speaking up on many issues in the bill we were marking up, ranging from support for joint training of social workers in medical schools to the impact of phasing out foreign medical graduates from inner-city residency programs. I had been fortunate to have spent two years in a medical school with close ties to a large medical center, and I had taught medical students, so I knew a bit about their concerns firsthand. As discussions progressed, I could learn, from people I respected, how particular legislative provisions might affect their programs and activities. Certainly I am no expert on medical education, but my knowing the problems from the inside helped make earlier academic preparation useful as I worked with my peers. After all, a policy—a deliberate set of actions aimed at achieving certain goals and objectives—seeks to bring about changes in a large-scale environment that consists of real institutions and real people. A very good way to make bad policy is to rely on theory or rational common sense while remaining ignorant of how things work in the real world.

Experience cannot substitute for critical thinking, though it is an important ingredient in the mixture of cognition and intuition that produces judgment. The administrator with a solid knowledge of the health system contributes to health policy that concerns hospitals and other institutions, financing and organization of services, health planning, and so on. The health care field is not altogether unique in the nation's domestic economy, but it is not entirely interchangeable with other sectors either. The health administrator on a policy staff is apt to know the peculiarities of the system up close. The network of contacts—people one can turn to for advice, information, and reactions—is very helpful, too. Like testimony from interest groups, advice

121

from respected colleagues in the field has to be filtered critically in light of the problems and constraints at hand. Once inside government, the old saw remains the best summary: "Where you stand depends on where you sit."[32]

By virtue of both training and experience, the health administrator is probably temperamentally suited to and certainly familiar with the slow and complicated process that characterizes institutional change. He or she has had to live with the politics of organizations, and thus probably tends toward pragmatic problem solving as a matter of day-to-day style. Most health administrators, too, have had experience in the frustrations and satisfactions of working with people of diverse backgrounds and interests. As noted, these attributes of patience and flexibility are essential for the policy analyst in government, too. And, health administrators, unlike most of their other colleagues in the policymaking arena, have been educated in public health to examine systematically health problems as they affect population groups. They can thus assess health policies with a strong sense of the common denominator.

Graduate training in the health field—even if it has followed job experience—seems to consolidate after some first-hand struggle and participation in the health care system. Thus, the new graduate, even one with an advanced degree in health policy, will probably contribute less to a policy position—and learn less from it—than a person who has had some seasoning. The greatest satisfaction can come from sharing knowledge that is based on one's skills and experience, and from knowing how it feels to be in the trenches.

Turning that argument around, I believe that there is a very real danger of growing stale and isolated, or increasingly dependent on secondhand reports from the front. As time pressures mount, judgments have to be taken, and sometimes people get sloppy or arrogant. The best antidote to this is probably a change of scene. In fact, most health policy analysts in government, regardless of their original profession, do just that. We are not exactly a restless lot, but many of us seem willing to turn our energies to various points in the health care system and to teaching and research communities, thus transferring our baggage of newly acquired knowledge and skills to the service of new settings and new tasks.[33]

It is hard to convey just how complex, richly textured, and unpredictable the political environment is, and how knotted the threads of the processes that make an impact on policy. After two years, I felt I was just beginning to learn, and more seasoned and senior analysts than this writer confirm their endless amazement at the serendipity of democracy. It may not be possible to see the river while swimming in its currents. Moreover, after leaving government health policy analysis for a time, the practitioner of that sometimes arcane art comes away with a sense not only of the limitations of government and of the constraints of democracy but also of what is possible, and how to achieve it. Returning to the health care system itself from the world of government health policy making, the former analyst has learned how and where to bring information to bear on future policy—how to continue to contribute to political life.

NOTES

[1]H. David Banta and Patricia Bauman, "Health Services Research and Health Policy." *Journal of Community Health* 2, no. 2, (Winter 1976): p. 123.

[2]I hope readers will not give undue significance to the pronouns "he," "his," etc., to indicate the third person singular. This current English usage happens to describe life on the Hill. Its 535 functionally equal members exempted Congress from the provisions of the Civil Rights Act, and so there are probably as many sets of personnel practices as there are members.

[3]Odin W. Anderson, "Influence of Social and Economic Research on Public Policy in the Health Field: A Review." *Milbank Memorial Fund Quarterly*, 50, 3 Part 2, 1966. pp. 11–48.

[4]Richard M. Titmuss, *Social Policy: An Introduction*. New York: Pantheon Books, 1974. p. 23.

[5]Lowell E. Bellin, "Googooland and New York City: Comparative Physiology of Two Health Departments." Unpublished manuscript, 1977. Bellin provides a convincing front-line account of the futility and danger of ignoring the democratic process.

[6]Allen Schicke's description of congressional use of analysis applies also to the executive branch, with the important difference that most major policies arise there, so that the supply of analysis is more regular: "Congress must function as a massive scanning machine, sucking in data and arguments from many sources and refining them into legislative material. In this role, Congress treats analysis much as it treats gossip, news, constituency mail, the local newspaper, etc. Everything is grist for the Congressional mill, and analysis enjoys no preferred position by virtue of its esteem in intellectual circles. The legislative product will be a compound of analysis and countless other types of input." From "The Supply and Demand for Analysis on Capitol Hill," in *U.S. Congress, A Compilation of Papers Prepared for the Commission on the Operation of the Senate*, 94th Congress, Second Session, Washington, D.C., 1976. pp. 72–85. Reprinted from *Policy Analysis* 2 (Spring 1976): pp. 215–34.

[7]Health policy analysis may thus be a career for relatively young people whose family responsibilities permit some job insecurity.

[8]Joseph L. Falkson, "Minor Skirmish in a Monumental Struggle: HEW's Analysis of Mental Health Services. *Policy Analysis* 2 (Winter 1976): pp. 93–119 (see especially p. 102). See also John Quarles, *Cleaning Up America: An Insider's View of the Environmental Protection Agency*. Boston: Houghton Mifflin Co., 1976. Quarles provides an excellent description not only of the commonly shared world view of his agency, but also of how that view conflicted with that of the White House and with those of other cabinet departments.

[9]Over 25,000 bills are introduced in Congress each year. Over 2,000 of them relate to health. They are referred to a particular committee (or sometimes referred jointly to more than one), and thence to a subcommittee in each House. Any member of Congress can introduce a bill on any subject. Only a small proportion receive hearings. Still fewer bills go through the further legislative process of markup in subcommittee; in committee; consideration by the full chamber; referral to House-Senate conference committee to reconcile differences; reconsideration of the compromise by both bodies; submission to the President. For a full description of the process, see U.S. Government Printing Office, *How Our Laws Are Made*. Washington, D.C., periodically updated. For a description of the process as it applies to health care, see H. David Banta, "The Federal Legislative Process and Health Care," in Jonas, Steven, et al., *Health Care Delivery in the United States*. New York: Springer Publishing Co., 1977.

[10]Senate Resolution 4, U.S. Senate, *Congressional Record*, January 4, 1927. There are many motives for reorganization, and it is often undertaken for its own sake, to reflect or create shifts in power, and so forth. For a lively discussion of what reorganization can and cannot do, see Harold Seidman, *Politics, Position, and Power: The Dynamics of Federal Organization*. New York: Oxford University Press, 1970.

[11]Patricia Bauman and H. David Banta, "The Congress and Policymaking for Prevention," *Preventive Medicine* 6 (1977): pp. 227–41. The authors consider how the committee system affects Congress's ability to deal with issues like prevention that, ideally, require policy integration. As cited in this reference, see also Lewis Dexter's discussion of the advantages of "creative redundancy," whereby a problem gets consideration from several diverse points of view.

[12]Aaron Wildavsky, *The Politics of the Budgetary Process*. Boston: Little, Brown and Co., 1974.

[13]In the Senate, the major committees that deal with health legislation are Human Resources for the Public Health Service Act (Public Health Service programs, FDA, NIH, etc.) and Finance for Medicare and Medicaid. Counterparts in the House are the Committees on Interstate and Foreign Commerce (Subcommittee on Health and Environment) and Ways and Means. In the House, however, the committees share jurisdiction over Part B of Medicare, since it is financed by general tax revenues; thus, the Committee on Interstate and Foreign Commerce oversees Medicaid, too. In both Houses of Congress the persistent split between financing and issues of organization and manpower impedes progress toward national health insurance and a planned system. Also in both Houses, the Appropriations subcommittees that deal with the HEW budget recommend spending levels for authorized programs, and of these 50 have considerable influence on health policy outcomes.

[14]R.F. Fenno, Jr., *Congressmen in Committees*. Boston: Little, Brown and Co., 1973.

[15]David E. Price, *Who Makes the Laws? Creativity and Power in Senate Committees*. Cambridge, Massachusetts: Schenkman, 1972.

[16]Nathan W. Polsby, "Strengthening Congress in National Policymaking." In *Congressional Behavior*, Nathan W. Polsby, ed. New York: Random House, 1971.

[17]Graham T. Allison, "Conceptual Models and the Cuban Missile Crisis," *American Political Science Review* 63, no. 3 (September 1969): pp. 689–719. Allison describes some predictable, functional attributes of organizational behavior.

[18]Rufus Miles, *The Department of Health, Education, and Welfare*. New York: Praeger Publishers, 1974; Stephen Strickland, *Politics, Science, and Dread Disease*. Cambridge: Harvard University Press, 1972; John Quarles, *Cleaning Up America: An Insider's View of the Environmental Protection Agency*, note 8.

[19]Hugo Heclo, "Bureaucratic Sabotage: How Civil Servants Undercut Presidential Appointees." *The Washington Post*, August 14, 1977, p. B-1.

[20]Joseph L. Falkson, *op. cit.* (note 8), pp. 102–103.

[21]David Mayhew, *Congress: The Electoral Connection*. New Haven: Yale University Press, 1974.

[22]The general public is certainly made up of constituents, but they rarely write about health policy issues; abortion and laetrile are notable exceptions. Most mail deals with specific problems, like costs for uncovered services under Medicare, or a transfer to an American medical school from a foreign one. This public communication is instructive about real problems in the system, and it may accordingly give rise to changes. It is neither organized nor vigorous, however.

[23]Harold S. Luft, "Benefit-Cost Analysis and Public Policy Implementation: From Normative to Positive Analysis." *Public Policy* 23, no. 4 (Fall 1976): pp. 437-62. See, especially, p. 447.

[24]A legislator's administrative assistant or other top personal staff person, in a role analogous to that of political experts in executive departments, often serves as a political filter, sifting ideas and issues put forth by the legislator's other staff, who are assigned to gain a special understanding of specific issues or to concentrate on the work of particular committees, to ensure that the member of Congress has a strong and consistent platform.

[25]E. Schattschneider, *The Semi-Sovereign People*. Hinsdale, Illinois: The Dryden Press, 1960.

[26]Stanley Karnow, "Non-Elected Power on Capitol Hill." *The Washington Post*, August 26, 1977. Karnow quotes Senator Thomas Morgan: "Morgan revealed the process,

perhaps too frankly for his colleagues, when he said: 'They are the ones who give us advice as to how to vote, and then we vote on their recommendations.' " Allen Schick, too, notes that staff provide congressional members with a broader reach that has become necessary as the entire purview of Congress and the executive branch has expanded to encompass a very wide range of national and foreign issues (though there is not necessarily any greater depth on any single issue). Schick, *op. cit.* (note 6).

[27]Bruce L.R. Smith, ed., *The New Political Economy: The Public Use of the Private Sector.* New York: Macmillan, 1974. See, especially, the Introduction.

[28]The scientific method, *per se,* is not always evident in all epidemiology courses as taught, but its principles govern in practice.

[29]Richard M. Titmuss, *op. cit.* (note 4), p. 59.

[30]P. Ellwood, "Uses of Data in Health Policy Formulation," oral presentation at the annual meetings of the Association of Teachers of Preventive Medicine, Chicago, November 16, 1975.

[31]H. David Banta and Patricia Bauman, *op. cit.* (note 1); Joseph L. Falkson, *op. cit.* (note 8); Harold S. Luft, *op. cit.* (note 23); Allen Schick, *op. cit.* (note 6).

[32]Harold Seidman, *op. cit.* (note 10), p. 20, attributes this remark to Rufus Miles, former Assistant Secretary for Administration, Department of Health, Education and Welfare.

[33]The policy-analysis world is seductive and small, its niches filled by a relatively close-knit group of Washington-based people (see above, pp. 20–21), together with analysts and researchers who fly into and out of the Capital from universities and other settings all over the country. Hence, there is not as much cross-fertilization between those who plan and those who do as I believe would be mutually beneficial. Many people find it hard to go back to smaller settings once they have been in some part of government.

11 As Private Consultant: Trailblazer or Hired Gun?

Arnold I. Kisch, M.D., M.P.H.

Information is costly. Useful advice is invaluable. The health administrator, no matter how capable or conscientious he or she may be, in whatever specialty, is hardly omniscient. The prudent health administrator or the board of the agency, therefore, periodically invites consultants from the outside to come into the shop, take a fresh look at the enterprise, help identify problems, and make recommendations to improve its operation. How useful is the consultant in these roles?

Arnold Kisch, a consultant and professor, explores the world of consulting in health administration in the next chapter. (L.E.B.)

Introduction

Some years ago, there appeared a Peanuts cartoon captioned, "The world is full of people anxious to serve in an advisory capacity." If this is true of the world in general, it is even more true of the field of health administration where, in recent decades, private consultants have made major inroads, appearing in a variety of settings and assuming an impressively large array of functions. This chapter will focus on the private consultant in health administration from several perspectives. First, it will discuss the evolving nature of the role. Second, it will present the areas of knowledge and the technical skills that appear most relevant to this profession. Third, it will discuss the need for private consultants in the field of health administration, and the moral dilemma posed by their utilization. Fourth, it will present some of the practical aspects one encounters when trying to earn a living as a private consultant in health administration; and finally, (perhaps unavoidably, since this is the arena of the author's personal experience), it will discuss the special situations one encounters when pursuing simultaneously the career of a private consultant and that of an academic. The chapter will, I hope, provide some insights and offer some points of reference to students who may themselves be contemplating a career in private consulting.

The Evolution of Private Consulting in Health Administration

Although private consultants have been playing a major role in health administration only in recent decades, there exists a long and honorable history of individual consultants whose contributions have had a major effect on the American health care system. In this regard, it should be noted that the first major systematic effort to upgrade the quality of American medicine began in 1910 with a report issued by the Carnegie Foundation and its consultant, Dr. Abraham Flexner.[1] Other examples of seminal reports produced by individual consultants can also be cited. There is, for example, the five-year study by the Committee on the Cost of Medical Care, which,

Arnold I. Kisch, M.D., M.P.H., is President of ARNO Associates, in Santa Monica, California.

under sponsorship of private foundations, used the services of a variety of experts to achieve a comprehensive analysis of the American health care system that still has relevance today.[2] Prominent academics, such as Dr. Roger Irving Lee of Harvard, were among the consultants who produced reports that were eventually issued by the Committee.[3] The tradition has been continued over the years. In 1945, for example, Yale University's Dr. Haven Emerson produced a report, *Local Health Units for the Nation*, which served as a model for the reorganization of health departments around the country.[4] Similarly, in the years 1962–1966, the National Commission on Community Health Services, using a large number of consultants (many from university faculties), produced a ten-volume report which provided a general blueprint for the delivery of community health services in the United States.[5] Many other similar examples can be cited.The value of work done by private consultants in health administration has long been recognized by government, even though this positive valuation has not always been openly acknowledged. Thus in 1946, a group of private citizens in Los Angeles County, concerned about the rapid local population growth and the strain that this would very likely place on existing hospital bed resources, hired a private consultant who developed a countywide hospital plan.[6] The plan identified twenty hospital service areas which coincided with business economic areas. When shortly thereafter the State of California sought to implement the Hill-Burton legislation for the first time, it was necessary to define hospital service areas throughout the state. For Los Angeles, the California State Department of Public Health and the Bureau of Hospitals merely adopted the boundaries that had been drawn earlier by the private consultant.

In time, this particular action came to illustrate both the advantages and the potential disadvantages inherent in using a private consultant to do the government's work in the area of health administration. In the short run, the hospital service areas outlined by the private consultant saved the government trouble and expense and provided a basis for allocating Hill-Burton funds in Los Angeles. In the long run, however, this quick acceptance of a private consultant's work, done to suit non-government sponsors with motivations of their own, proved problematic. After the Watts riots of 1965, the government of California reassessed for the first time the equity of the hospital service areas that it had adopted some twenty years before, and found that approximately 300,000 residents of Los Angeles in effect had no ready access to acute care general hospitals. Their need for hospital beds was masked by the manner in which the hospital service area boundaries had been drawn.[7] The service area boundaries were subsequently redrawn. Only then did it become possible to justify funding for the construction of a new hospital to serve the poor people of Los Angeles. Such problems notwithstanding, private consultants have been used increasingly in the various aspects of health administration where government (federal, state, and local) has a responsibility. There are several reasons for this increase in utilization:

1. The private consultant is frequently viewed as bringing a fresh perspective to the matters under consideration, perhaps a different perspective from that of government employees who are expected to be more traditional in their points of view.
2. The use of a consultant is often regarded as a cost-effective way to get a job done, since it neither requires taking existing government employees away from their assigned tasks, nor does it commit the government to the hiring of new full-time personnel.
3. The use of a private consultant may be a means of introducing a new planning or administration technique. The hope here is that the new technique may provide a breakthrough in helping to solve problems which have long plagued the program in question.
4. An unwritten code states that the private consultant is more likely to get the job done (and do it well) than is a government employee with civil service tenure. Since full-time government employees have rarely, if ever, been given the

incentives to produce that are routinely granted to the consultant, the truth of this concept cannot be determined. Whatever its origins, however, the myth is vigorously encouraged by the consultants.

Even where the law does not specifically require the use of consultants, government is increasingly involving them in its health care programs. The scope of tasks assigned to consultants by federal, state, and local government agencies is very broad. For example, in the past decade consultants were hired to train consumers to function on the Boards of Neighborhood Health Centers established under programs funded by the Federal Office of Economic Opportunity. At the present time numerous requests for proposals by the federal government seek to involve private consultants in the task of developing technical assistance materials for the state and local planning agencies set up under the National Health Planning and Resources Development Act of 1974 (P.L.93–641).

Private consultants are being called upon more and more often to assist the government even in drafting legislation and implementing regulations. One example here will illustrate a fairly common phenomenon. P.L. 93–641 requires designated planning agencies to assess the health status of the population and to measure the impact which the health care delivery system is having on that health status. After P.L. 93–641 was enacted, it became apparent that the technology for carrying out these two mandated functions was largely missing, that in fact the very definition of health status was imprecise to the point that it was difficult if not impossible to render operational. The remedy adopted by the federal government to alleviate this problem involved contracting with a number of private consultants to develop retrospectively the definitions and technology which had erroneously been thought to exist, and which had been incorporated into the law. It has become routine practice to hire private consultants to evaluate established government health care programs. Such evaluations deal with many aspects of program operation, including quality of care, cost, and effectiveness. Several private consulting firms are today specializing in this type of work. The steady flow of government monies for this purpose has provided the financial underpinning for a thriving industry.

The private sector has been following the government's lead; its use of consultants has become an almost indispensable ingredient in the delivery of health care services. Private industry frequently hires consultants to interpret government regulations in the area of health administration. To give but one example of this, certificate-of-need legislation has created an entire new market for consultants who are able to interpret the nuances of the legislation and its implementing regulations to private health care providers interested in expanding their physical plants.

Not infrequently, the consultants hired to assist private providers in dealing with government regulations are the same consultants who worked for the government in developing the regulations in the first place. The free-lance nature of the consultant role, and since, as a former aide to government, the consultant may possess the most detailed inner knowledge of the law in question, make him or her an ideal partner for private providers striving to conduct business within the bounds of a complicated new health law. This situation is discussed more fully in a later section on the ethics of private consulting.

The expanding role assigned to consultants in health care administration and the prosperity of individual consultants and consulting firms have brought large corporations into the field as well. Recent years have witnessed the buying up of a number of health care consulting firms by big, diversified corporations. The consulting firm often continues to operate under its original name while the new corporate owner maintains a low profile in the operation of the consulting business. However, this has not always been the case. For example, in the very recent past, the nation's principal accounting firms began to move aggressively into the field of health care consultation. The entrée here has been through auditing. The accounting firm, having established a track record for auditing a particular hospital or health plan, suggests next that it provide consultation in the area of master planning, quality assurance, or the obtaining of a certificate of need. With their nationwide connections and ability to provide both accounting and consulting services, these large firms have been able to gain a significant foothold in the field of health care consultation in a relatively short time.

Owners of hospital chains (whether proprietary or not for profit) have also recently been offering consulting services to other, unaffiliated institutions. These consulting firms have as their main credentials the expertise gained within their own hospital chains and the financial backing which those chains can provide in the first period of independent existence. The growth of these consulting firms has, by and large, been less assured than that of firms connected with the major accounting corporations or other large, diversified business enterprises.

Architectural firms and law firms have also been branching out into the field of health care consultation. In the case of architectural firms, the emphasis has tended to be on institutional planning—designing an appropriate mission to go with a set of buildings. Law firms, by contrast, have concentrated more on assisting providers in the process of dealing with obstacles posed by laws and government regulations.

Whatever the cause, recent years have witnessed a rapid, dynamic growth in the area of private consultation for health administration. Growth has been so rapid, in fact, that it may conceivably become desirable in the future to hire a consultant to look into the optimal role of consultants in this field. It would be appropriate, after this introduction, to take a closer look next at the array of knowledge and skills which consultants bring to bear in the area of health administration.

Knowledge and Skills Required of the Consultant

Many and varied types of expertise are sought in health administration consulting. It is unlikely that any one person's knowledge could ever encompass them all. Moreover, health care consultants are becoming more and more specialized, mirroring the general trend among health care providers. A partial list of the range of desired knowledge and technical skills includes the following: accounting, communication, community organization, cost-benefit analysis, data analysis, education, facilities design, finance, information systems, legal and legislative aspects of health care delivery, marketing, quality assurance, rate setting, systems analysis, and survey design.

A student planning to undertake a career in health administration consulting should make an effort to acquire thorough knowledge in one or more of these areas. All of them are in demand. The only requirement is that one's knowledge be well founded in theory, yet tempered with enough field experience to permit an understanding of the realistic constraints involved in applying theory to practice. Convincing a potential client of one's skill is a further necessary ingredient for success as a consultant. This aspect is discussed more fully below.

The two most likely places to receive training in the designated areas are a school of public health or a school of business administration. The most sought-after credentials for entry level health administration consultants are the M.B.A. or the M.P.H. Higher levels of consultation responsibility are being reserved more and more often for those with doctoral degrees. Such degrees may be in a variety of related fields such as public health, business, economics, public administration, and so forth.

One also finds persons with M.D., D.D.S., or J.D. degrees working as consultants in the field of health administration. These persons, however, are beginning to acquire secondary M.P.H. degrees, since it is becoming recognized that merely going to medical school, dental school, or law school does not provide to a sufficient degree the skills sought in a health administration consultant.

At schools of public health and business administration one now can find programs which allow students to acquire an interdepartmental type of education. Here the object is to blend traditional management and health skills. Such a blend is particularly relevant to the field of consultation in health administration. At several schools today a combined M.B.A.–M.P.H. degree is offered, formally recognizing this pattern of education.

Other educational programs in fields such as law, architecture, and economics are also beginning to require students interested in health applications to combine education programs either by attending a number of health courses while getting their basic degrees, or by taking a special master's degree in public health after completing their studies in the areas of their primary interest. Less frequently one sees persons with a degree such as a J.D. taking a master's degree in business administration in preparation for work as a consultant in health administration. It seems well recognized that, for those lacking formal training in health care, an M.P.H. or its equivalent is the necessary prerequisite for work in the area of health administration.

The opportunities for acquiring interdisciplinary training in preparation for work in the field of health administration are increasing. Similarly, interest on the part of students to take such programs appears to be on the rise. While it is hard to advise students in general about an optimal combination for a joint degree, the overall favorites at this time among potential employers of health administration consultants seem to be the health-administration, health-law, and health-economics combinations.

The greatest pleasure in working as a consultant, I think, comes from functioning in an independent capacity, bringing to bear one's own expertise in solving a client's problem. It is clear, however, that a student fresh out of school, whatever the educational background, will not be prepared to function as a consultant at this level for some time. It is necessary first to gain field experience and seasoning, often over a period of years and in a variety of settings. Some will prefer to get this experience in an agency or in an institutional setting. Others will prefer to get it as a junior member of a consulting firm. While both routes can lead ultimately to the desired goal of a career as an independent consultant, it seems preferable to choose a path that allows for spending some time in a position with direct line administrative responsibility. Those who go from school directly to employment with a consulting firm run the risk of giving consultant advice which runs counter to the simple, practical operational constraints that are of common knowledge to administrators in the field—the very ones perhaps who have engaged the consultant. This failing can prove to be a fatal flaw, wholly undermining the consultant's effectiveness. The only reliable antidote is for the health administration consultant to have first-hand administrative knowledge. This can be acquired only one way—by spending some portion of one's professional career functioning as an administrator at an agency, in an institution, or within the government.

The Ethics of Private Consultation

Given the current situation in health administration, in which consultants are being employed by both the government and the private sector, and where individuals are flocking to careers in the field of private consultation, it seems pointless to question whether there is in fact a need for private consultants. The obvious perceived need has several dimensions.

First, it is simply too difficult and too expensive for most health care organizations (or even the government) to have available among their employees at all times the great variety of skills outlined above, any of which may be required to solve problems which may arise in the organization from time to time.

Second, the skills needed to solve a particular problem in the organization are in many cases highly technical and require a knowledge of theory best developed by those who have the opportunity to work full-time at acquiring their specialized knowledge, together with the opportunity to interact with other theoreticians. Such an opportunity is rarely available in a product-oriented organizational setting.

Third, it is frequently desirable to bring an outsider into an established situation with the hope of obtaining a fresh point of view on a chronic, vexing problem. The consultant is an obvious choice for this role.

131

Finally, it is possible, through the simultaneous employment of several consultants on related projects, for an organization to develop alternative strategies for overcoming difficult operational problems. Employing the overlapping consultants has been used with success in government agencies. Carefully evaluating the relative benefits of the alternative approaches can prove to be an effective way to discover the optimal solution to complicated problems, in health administration as well as in other enterprises.

Granted, then, that the private consultant does fill a real, even a multidimensional need in the area of health administration, the question still remains whether the consultant comes upon the scene as a trailblazer or as a hired gun. In this regard, both the consultant and his or her employer must be aware that there is an inherent moral dilemma in the situation. Both must make a conscientious effort to behave in a responsible manner. To recognize the fact that material released in the name of the government may in fact have been written by a private consultant, or that a government consultant who has worked closely in drafting a law may later be hired by private interests to assist in their functioning at the margin of that same law and its regulations, is not in itself cause for alarm. However, certain elements in such situations clearly lend themselves to abuse by unscrupulous or careless persons.

In theory, the private consultant is brought in as a highly trained and independent thinker who is possessed of some special skills. In practice, it is at all times clear to the consultant that his or her professional success depends upon pleasing the client. On the other side, the client (often an individual or a small group of individuals within a larger organization) may view the hiring of a consultant as an opportunity to prevail in a situation where several points of view are vying with each other. While selecting a particular consultant, or developing the specifics of the work contract with the consultant, the client has an opportunity to exert influence over the consultant, leading away from the exercise of independence of thought. Ultimately, this can result in a less than competent, or perhaps even less than honest, consulting report, one which mirrors the wishes of the client rather than the best judgment of the expert consultant.

It is very hard to avoid this moral dilemma, because the consultant has no official status and ultimately is responsible only to the person signing the contract with him or her. Nor is the consultant readily made accountable for the quality of work delivered. He or she has no guarantee that the product delivered will be used in its entirety. One of the most frustrating situations a consultant encounters is seeing partial implementation of one's recommendations when such action may not only be inappropriate but also may contradict the thrust of the report in its entirety. Only in cases where the consultant's name is attached to the product (by no means a universal occurrence) does he or she acquire the right to challenge the client and attempt to straighten the record. To exercise this right, however, is a highly risky procedure. A consultant who publicly takes issue with his client is very likely to hurt his or her prospects for acquiring future business.

While it may be public knowledge that a consultant has been brought in to some situation, the exact details of the contract drawn up with the consultant are rarely made public. Even where these details are known, there is almost no way to assess the degree to which the consultant has been permitted to act in an independent fashion. Nor is it possible to assess accurately whether the consultant's recommendations have been released in the full context in which they were presented to the client.

Beyond these moral considerations, consultants should be further concerned for what might be called the cross-pollination effect of their services. Moving from assignment to assignment, consultants invariably pick up inside knowledge which can be brought to bear in future projects. Consultants can be constrained from revealing information obtained through medical records or other sensitive data sources, but there is no way to keep them from using the knowledge of the inner workings of an organization which they acquired as a natural by-product of working in a particular setting. In a parallel situation, there are regulations which constrain a government employee from working for a private company which has been contracting with the government for a specified period of time after the employee leaves government service. However, a private consultant cannot be similarly constrained. This, too, raises the possibility that the private consultant may function as a hired gun. Working inside government, for example, a consultant can learn the most intimate ins and outs of a piece of health legislation and also the personal philosophy of those government officials charged with implementing the law. The same consultant may soon after be engaged to work for clients whose basic purpose is to avoid obeying the intent of the particular legislation. The consultant, an unlicensed freelancer, is subject in this situation to temptations that may be impossible to resist.

There are no ready or easy solutions to the moral problems that have been posed here. The nature of a consultant's work is piecemeal. It is all too easy, then, for all concerned to avoid focusing on the work occupied by an individual consultation within the larger framework of the dynamics of a health administration situation.

The consultant's role within health administration must be better defined and more clearly recognized by the public if safeguards are to be constructed to avoid its possible corruption. As things now stand, the consultant—a knowledgeable person with skills to sell—cannot be asked to assume responsibility if his or her product eventually is used for less than benign purposes. The very nature of consulting work at present contributes to this problem, and it is the nature of that work which will concern us next.

The Consultant's Working Environment

The life of a private consultant is a precarious one, including moments of feast and famine. When numerous requests for proposals are issued which appear to be in the area of the consultant's knowledge or skills, he or she must respond to a number of them. Herein lies the potential for the first problem. Sometimes one hits a dry period. No contracts are won even though many proposals are written by the consulting firm. It is then necessary to lay off employees and generally cut back all expenses. On the other hand, there are times when several contracts are won all at once, giving the firm more work than had been anticipated. It is then necessary to hire additional employees, often in a hurry, with insufficient time to select fully qualified personnel.

Except in larger, well-established consulting firms with substantial resources, the feast and famine cycle of contract awards makes orderly long-range planning very difficult for consultants. The consulting field is highly competitive. One never has the luxury of simply working on a contract and enjoying it. The consultant must always have an eye toward the future, scouting for new business even while fulfilling work under existing contracts. The consultant hopes that, in time, current work will lead to repeat business. Such repeat business will more likely come directly to the consulting firm without involving competitive bids. It may also arrive in a manner that can be scheduled more conveniently. It is dangerous, however, for a consulting firm to rely too heavily on repeat customers at the expense of seeking new clients. The search for new clients consumes time and energy and money, but it is necessary work at all times.

Like any business, a consulting firm does best at a time when it is growing. The consulting firm relies in large measure, however, on selling the expertise of its individual members. There probably exists an ideal caseload, at which point the experts in the consulting firm are most able to assist clients in an efficient manner. However, to achieve exactly this level of work and to hold it steadily over time is extremely difficult. The successful company may grow too large by overextending its employees or by hiring people who may not be as qualified as the initial consultant group. Alternatively, the company may grow too slowly, and lose its competitive edge, together with the services of its best consultants. Some highly specialized consulting firms seem able to avoid this dilemma. For most, however, it is a very serious problem. Any business turned away represents a hazard to a firm's reputation as a capable concern. Yet a firm may well reach a point where its personnel feel saturated for a period of six or eight months. They must then decide whether to deny potential clients or to expand, perhaps at a risk of overextending themselves. Thus, the consulting firms that might be most attractive to a client—relatively small firms offering the services of experts with specific skills at low overhead cost—have a hard time staying in business. Alternative firms—larger, financially more secure, always able to accept new clients—may be far less adaptable to the clients' needs, much more expensive, and oriented toward doing business the company's way. Yet, these firms may prove to be more viable over time.

The private consultant attempting to operate his or her own firm—perhaps working jointly with a small group of colleagues or less formally trained assistants—is forever being challenged by potential clients on grounds of the firm's stability. The client is likely to ask, "What happens if you fall dead in the street tomorrow?" or, "Do you have access to a major computing facility?" It seems pointless to advise the potential client that even large firms lack a large assortment of thoroughly qualified individuals, that in any setting the death of any one senior person on a project will seriously affect the outcome. It also seems pointless to tell the client that the actual computer needs will not require facilities other than those already available to the small consulting firm. Too often the client wants a demonstration of size to offset his or her own insecurity at having to hire a consultant in the first place.

Another practical aspect in the life of a private consultant is the constant presence of very short deadlines. The operational motto of the army, which used to be "Hurry up and wait," applies to the world of the private consultant. Every proposal request seems to come with no more than a thirty-day deadline. This means that, from the time one actually sees a request until the finished proposal must go in the mail, one may have no more than two to three weeks. In that brief period of time, the consultant is expected to become familiar with the underlying problem, learn in some detail the constraints within which the client is dealing with the problem, and come up with a realistic work plan by which the client can be given the assistance requested and a budget figure to match. Then a concise, readable proposal must be written, typed, duplicated, and mailed. This is a very tall order indeed.

The firm's usual procedure for dealing with this limit is to develop a less than thorough proposal. The hope is that after a contract is acquired, there will be time to flesh out the details. Alternatively, the consulting firm may apply to the given situation a methodology that it has already used in a previous, perhaps related project. However, such decisions cast doubt on the quality of the report that will eventually result from the contract.

Not only are the deadlines attached to requests for proposals unreasonably tight, but also no money is usually offered for the task of preparing a proposal. The consultant, however, may incur considerable expense in preparing to write an intelligent proposal. For example, he or she may need to visit a proposed project site. Almost invariably, he or she will need to research the literature, or to prepare charts or other graphics to illustrate a proposal. The fact that responses to proposals must be made as a sideline to work on projects already in house contributes to the sloppy thinking that often goes into these documents. Viewed as a gamble by the firm, the proposals rarely get the best efforts of the consultant staff. When a contract is subsequently awarded, the work plan under the project is usually constrained in its time frame as well. It becomes difficult at this point to do the conceptual work that should have been done at the time the proposal was prepared in the first place. It seems evident that consultants would do consistently better work if they were given adequate resources and time to develop well considered proposals. It seems unlikely, however, that such a situation will develop in the near future.

Where repeat business is involved, it is more likely that the client will come to a preselected consultant and develop with him or her a careful work proposal. This is an ideal situation, allowing for a good deal of constructive interchange at the important moment when the proposal is conceptualized. This situation is, however, more the exception than the rule. More commonly, proposals are put together in the hustle and bustle of competitive bidding.

Another problem faced by consultants in health administration is that clients frequently do not reveal the amount of money they wish to spend for the project at hand. The thinking here seems to be that if the sum of money available were made known, no proposals would come in for less than this amount, and that by being secretive one can save money by achieving low bids. This may well be true. On the other hand, from the consultant's point of view, it would be immensely helpful to know the amount of money the client has to spend at the outset. If the sum offered turned out to be too little to make a proposal feasible from the consultant's perspective, the consultant might be spared the trouble of developing a meaningful proposal. Alternatively, given the knowledge of the sum which the prospective client has to spend, it would be possible for the consultant to fashion a proposal offering the most innovative or effective consultation design which can be devised within the budget constraints.

Lacking knowledge of the amount of money in question, consultants concentrate rather on proposing to spend as little as possible. If very inexperienced, the consultant, guessing in the dark, may seriously underbid, and produce a low budget figure which the client in turn may buy, not realizing that the figure is so low that it is impossible for a good product to be developed. The client in such a situation may reject an alternative proposal by another consultant which, while somewhat more expensive, may be more realistic as far as giving the consultation the desired product. Later, it may be necessary for the client to pay additional funds to the low bidding consultant, or face the possibility of accepting a substandard product.

For some time the federal government has recognized this problem. In putting out its requests for proposals, it usually assigns to the project a given number of man years. This provides the consultant bidding on the proposal with a rough estimate from which to develop a cost projection. It seems unfortunate that others are not routinely following the government's practice in this regard.

Consultants in health administration operate as individuals, partnerships, or corporations. If they operate as corporations they may choose the for profit or not for profit form of organization. Certain types of government funding are awarded only to not for profit corporations. It is largely for this reason that some health administration consulting firms have chosen to organize on this basis. There are, however, relatively few penalties for operating as a for profit corporation, while the complications of doing business are greater in the not for profit mode. Today, with the government moving away from grants and towards contracts in awarding health monies, it is becoming less important for a consulting firm to organize on a not for profit basis.

Organizing as a solo consultant or as a partnership involves the risk to the consultant of unlimited personal liability and fails to provide the client with the security of dealing with an entity that could survive if an individual consultant did not. For this reason, even though there are expenses and some technical complications involved in incorporating, it seems desirable for a consulting firm to incorporate if it wishes seriously to pursue business over an extended period of time.

It is almost impossible to estimate the total number of consulting firms active in the field of health administration today. As has already been discussed, these firms assume many forms, ranging all the way from large multidimensional corporations to individuals working out of their private homes. There is no licensing or accrediting body to make a count of consultants in health administration. Further, in many of the smaller consulting firms, individual consultants are active on a part-time basis only. However, although the yellow pages of the telephone book may contain no listing for health administration consultants, numerous individuals and corporations around the country are consulting in health administration. Health administration consultants tend to cluster in certain locations (Washington, D.C., New York City, the West

Coast), but they are also found in most major cities and in a good many middle-sized communities.

Within the ranks of health administration consultants must be counted a sizable number of academics, professors who supplement their university salaries by consulting in the outside world. It is to this group of professionals and the constraints under which they function that attention will now be devoted.

The Academic-Consultant

It is not really surprising to find academics actively engaged in the field of health administration consulting. Traditionally, professors have laboratories or libraries on the university campus in which they pursue knowledge in their chosen fields. The product of this pursuit is scholarly papers, which eventually elicit recognition from the writer's peers.

However, those who teach health administration and such related disciplines as management, law, architecture, or geography, must ignore the traditional patterns of an academic career. For this group of academics, the real world situation *is* the laboratory. Libraries may offer some insights into relevant philosophy and technical skills, but they do not provide the bases for solving the problems that need to be solved in these practice-oriented fields. Success in these areas is measured more in terms of real life problems solved in the field than in terms of publications, speeches, or even prizes.

A professor of health administration who stays within the confines of the university runs the risk of losing touch with the field altogether. Each involvement with problems in the outside world, on the other hand, offers not only the chance to maintain practice skills but also the possibility of creating a situation where students can be brought to learn the skills of their chosen profession.

Not only professional motives draw professors into the field to solve health administration problems; economic motives function also. Involvement with the practical problems in the outside world provides a chance to supplement modest academic salaries. If that were not enough, there is also the chance to travel to new surroundings as an honored guest freely dispensing advice (and being listened to!). This is an ego booster that professors, tired of being less than fully appreciated on their home campuses, find very hard to resist. Small wonder, then, that academics are increasingly found to be stepping off campus to function as private consultants in health administration.

The academic-consultant serves within a range of possible roles. Some function in a part-time, individual capacity, dispensing ad hoc advice as it is requested. Others function as regular part-time employees, spending set periods of time each week or each month consulting in some particular setting. Occasionally, the academic will take a sabbatical leave and extend this part-time consulting role into a full-time function for some extended period of time.

Academics have also begun recently to appear in the health administration consulting arena as contractors. Sometimes as individuals, sometimes as partnerships, and sometimes as small corporations, academics are actually competing with established consulting firms for business. Academics who succeed in this regard frequently leave the university and shift their activities over completely to the private consulting sector.

The academic-consultant contributes distinct opportunities, together with distinct problems, to the field. On the positive side, the academic often brings the intimate knowledge of theory and skills he or she has developed as a teacher or researcher. Functioning on the university campus, the academic has a chance to broaden his or her knowledge and to refine it in the arena of give and take discussions with colleagues and students. Generally, the academic is articulate and can present his or her views in writing as well. The academic generally provides clients with the advantage of a relatively low price tag and the prestige of a name that has appeared in print and to which is appended a string of academic degrees.

The problems presented by the academic-consultant are not insignificant, however. For example, one can question the relevance of the academic viewpoint in many practical situations. It is by no means given that the academic serving as a consultant will understand the realities of field work. In the area of health administration, field conditions may vary distressingly from the theoretical constraints envisioned in the classroom. Not every academic can bridge this gap with ease.

There is also a concern about the availability and commitment of the academic-consultant. Especially when functioning as a part-time consultant, there is always the danger that the academic will withdraw to the safety of the university environment should the going get rough. There is very little that a consulting firm can do to hold on to a tenured professor who has suddenly decided to shift his or her focus back to the university campus right in the middle of a project.

If successful, the academic-consultant faces problems encountered by any small businessman—growing without exceeding his or her capacity. This can prove to be a particularly vexing problem for the academic-consultant. It was probably the chance to work in the field solving real life problems that attracted the academic to consulting. Now he or she finds that successful completion of consulting work leads to opportunities to do related work perhaps even more exciting or challenging than the original. Yet, he cannot respond to all requests, and recognizes that in each refusal lies the danger of destroying the momentum that has built up behind his budding consulting practice. A non-academic would likely resolve such a dilemma by expanding his or her firm's capacity. The academic-consultant generally lacks the capacity to respond to increased demands in this manner.

Even when holding growth within bounds, the academic-consultant may find that time devoted to consultation begins to detract from time devoted to research, teaching, and publication. Consultations come with short, specific deadlines. Faced with such pressures, one sometimes finds it easier to let the less highly structured academic deadlines slip by and to sacrifice one's availability to students than to fall behind on the consulting commitments.

Established consulting firms are not delighted when professors, working out of the safe environment of the university, appear in the field to compete for contracts. However, in the area of health administration, established consulting firms may be a good training site for students. When the professor becomes a competitor, it may undermine the good will which allows students access to the established consulting firms.

For those professors who can strike a proper balance between demands of the academic world and the demands of the consulting field, the role of the academic-consultant may be an ideal career situation. It affords all the excitement, the challenge, and the reward of the consulting field while providing the opportunity to renew one's expertise and energies on a regular basis. It also offers a safety net against the cyclical nature of the small consulting firm (the dry spells between contracts can be spent in mental refreshment and relaxation). Certain hazards are present, to be sure. One must learn to live with pressure, to budget one's time frugally, and to live with schedules that call for irregular hours and a good bit of travel.

To the successful academic-consultant, however, come a variety of very real rewards, such as the sense of knowing how to practice what one teaches, of being relevant in the real world as well as on campus. There is the fun of being invited to grapple with complex problems on behalf of a client who needs a practical solution. There is the opportunity to go into the field with one's best students—to give these bright minds a first exposure to field work and to watch the growth that the student achieves under such stimulus. There is the further opportunity to learn by getting close to people whom one would not usually meet on a university campus, people who are in practice the important movers and doers in the field of health administration. (I am here referring not only to elected officials but also to people from the business and management communities who daily run the enterprises about which academics teach in courses on health administration.) Finally, there is the unadulterated joy of realizing that one has achieved the Peanuts ideal in one's career: to be functionally one of the people who are privileged to serve in an advisory capacity (being paid real money to give advice). Consultants who are not academics may also share this pleasure, but to the academic-consultant comes the added joy of knowing that one will regularly have an audience of bright young students with whom he or she can share the insights gained in the field, and perhaps even the chance to write one's impressions for a chapter in a textbook. What more can one ask of a career?

NOTES

[1] A. Flexner, *Medical Education in the United States and Canada*. New York: The Carnegie Foundation for the Advancement of Teaching, 1910.

[2] The 28-volume final report was summarized in a single volume: *Medical Care for the American People, the Final Report of the Committee on the Costs of Medical Care, adopted October 31, 1932*. Chicago: University of Chicago Press, 1932.

[3] R.I. Lee, and L.W. Jones. *The Fundamentals of Good Medical Care*. Chicago: The University of Chicago Press, 1933.

[4] H. Emerson, *Local Health Units for the Nation. A Report for the American Public Health Association, Committee on Administrative Practice, Subcmmittee on Local Health Units*. New York: The Commonwealth Fund, 1945.

[5] The ten-volume report was summarized in the following volume: *Health Is a Community Affair, Report of the National Commission on Community Health Services*. Cambridge: Harvard University Press, 1967.

[6] J.A. Hamilton, *A Hospital Plan for Los Angeles County, Report to the Sponsoring Committee*. 1946.

[7] A.J. Viseltear, A.I. Kisch, and M.I. Roemer, *The Watts Hospital: A Health Facility Is Planned for a Metropolitan Slum Area*. Medical Care Administration, Case Study No. 5, U.S. Department of Health, Education and Welfare, Public Health Service, 1967.

The Minority Person as Health Administrator: From Token to Participant?

12

Haynes Rice, M.B.A., F.A.C.H.A.

Spokespeople from the variegated work settings of health administration have described their activities in independent chapters. In health service facilities health administrators, in their role as manager, expedite the work of clinicians to help alleviate the indelicacies that result from physiologic and behavioral dysfunction. This book would be incomplete if we failed to confront the obscene social indelicacy of racial and religious prejudice, operative in health administration itself. The problem is not trivial.

Haynes Rice, an experienced black health administrator and an activist in recruiting and educating minority health administrators, describes what has been accomplished—and what remains to be done. (L.E.B.)

In an interview with *Newsweek* Magazine the controversial Black comedian Richard Pryor commented, "I often have this dream: I'm in a beautiful grassy field surrounded by beautiful people and in the middle is an airplane. It's going to Heaven taking all the people there. I'm there too and I begin to look around and realize all the people are very pretty but they're White. So I decide I don't want to go to Heaven if there's not gonna be no Niggers there."[1]

Mr. Pryor's observation applies equally to the boards of directors meetings or executive staff meetings of the nation's health care institutions and associations. Black men and women are absent at these deliberations. There is but a single Black administrator among the nation's 7,700 hospitals whose patient mix is less than 50 percent Black or other minority group. As for women? Except for those representing religious orders, both White and Black women have been excluded from management positions other than those administering nursing departments. Women have a better chance for employment in health planning agencies, health associations, and consulting firms. But, even there, they can generally count on being hired primarily as administrative assistants. In 1977, neither Blacks nor women, except for one representing a religious order, served on the board of directors of the American Hospital Association.

Relatively little empirical data on minority health administrators exist.[2] This chapter proposes to examine some programs and other factors associated with the career patterns and mobility of minority health service administrators.

White health professionals often find it hard to relate transculturally to the medical and psychosocial needs of the Black, Puerto Rican, Mexican-American, Amerindian, and poor minority consumers of health care. Minority consumers who encounter flagrant insensitivity come to suspect even some of the well-intended actions of Whites. They may view such decisions as manifestations of White vindictiveness, greed for power, and a subtle devastating racism. I made this unflattering observation in an article called "To Cure Racism,"[3] and the observation still holds. Although

Haynes Rice, M.B.A., F.A.C.H.A. is Executive Director, Howard University Hospital, Washington, D.C.

minority health manpower has increased in the areas of administration and planning, opportunities are still few.[4] Currently only 4,731 minority people are counted among the nation's 84,461 health administrators.[5] To be sure, there has been moderate improvement in minority entry-level employment in the field of health services administration. Nevertheless, minority managerial professionals find their employment situations limited mostly to (1) tax-supported institutions, (2) Black institutions, (3) outpatient ambulatory care, and (4) community relations offices in voluntary hospitals.[6]

Health care delivery of acceptable quality to the minority community has always carried public health and political implications. The Flexner Report of 1910 addressed the issue of providing health care to Black people. Flexner's remarks still have pertinence today to minority people considering a career in health administration. Under the title "The Medical Education of the Negro," Dr. Flexner commented:

The medical care of the Negro race will never be wholly left to Negro physicians; nevertheless, if the Negro can be brought to feel a sharp responsibility for his people, the outlook for their mental and moral improvement will be drastically heightened. The practice of the Negro doctor will be limited to his own race, which in its turn will be cared for better by good Negro physicians than by poor White ones. But the physical well-being of the Negro is not only of moment to the Negro himself. Ten million of them live in close contact with sixty million Whites.[7]

Dr. Flexner emphasized that the Negro physician must be educated not only for his own sake or exclusively for the sake of his Black patients. Of obvious importance was the fact that the Negro patient suffered from hookworm and tuberculosis that could be transmitted to his White neighbors. The 1910 report recommended closing five of the seven Negro medical schools: (1) Flint Medical College, New Orleans, Louisiana, (2) Leonard Medical School, Raleigh, North Carolina, (3) Knoxville Medical College, Knoxville, Tennessee, (4) Medical Department of the University of West Tennessee, Memphis, Tennessee, and (5) National Medical College, Louisville, Kentucky. The report supported keeping two medical schools open: (1) Meharry Medical College, Nashville, Tennessee, and (2) Howard University Medical College, Washington, D.C. The report argued that Meharry at Nashville and Howard at Washington, D.C., were worth developing and that it would be wise to concentrate available efforts upon them.[8] It is not surprising that programs in health service administration were later developed to complement medical education at the same two institutions, Meharry Medical College and Howard University.

Meharry Program in Health Administration

Meharry Medical College Division of Health Care Administration and Planning is a cooperative educational venture operated by a consortium of three predominantly Black neighboring institutions in Nashville, Fisk University, Tennessee State University, and Meharry Medical College. In September, 1972, the Division began its training of middle-level health administrators and planners with seventeen students enrolled.[9] The student body was composed of twelve Blacks and five Mexican-Americans.[10]

Only three Black educational institutions offer degree programs in health administration or its equivalent; a Black student may seek the baccalaureate degree at Meharry Medical College and North Carolina Central University and the master's degree at Howard University.[11] Recently Meharry began a master's degree program also. At Howard University concentration in hospital administration leads to the M.B.A. degree, while concentration in health services administration leads to the M.P.A.

Programs for Minority Student Recruitment and Support

The National Association of Health Services Executives (NAHSE) was founded in 1968 at the annual meeting of the American Health Congress in Atlantic City, New Jersey. The late Whitney M. Young, keynote speaker at the Congress, challenged a group of predominantly Black health executives to organize and use their resources to improve health care for the poor of this country. NAHSE chapters have since been established in New York City, Chicago, Washington, D.C.-Baltimore, Nashville, Detroit, St. Louis, Kansas City, Kansas and Columbus, Ohio. The president of NAHSE is Bernard Dickens, whose office is at 2231 S. Western Avenue, Los Angeles, California 90018.

Summer Internships

Several initiatives have increased the number of minority students enrolled in graduate programs in health administration. Shortly after its founding in 1968, the National Association of Health Services Executives proposed to the Association of University Programs in Health Administration (then Hospital Administration) (AUPHA) that both collaboratively develop a career visibility program aimed at directing minority students into the health administration profession.[12] Two years later, in 1970, a pilot program designed to expose undergraduate students to health administration through summer internships began in Baltimore and New York. At the end of the first summer of the program 70 percent (25 out of 36) of the participants identified health administration as a career objective.[13] Since then the National Work-Study Recruitment Program in Health Administration for Minority Group Students has continued to encourage minority undergraduates to pursue careers in health administration. The students spend the summer in a hospital or other health care facility under the supervision of a health care administrator. Supplementing this apprenticeship are seminars and workshops dealing with relevant issues in the current health delivery system. Academic counseling is also provided.

In 1974, funding from the Health Resources Administration's Office of Health Resources Opportunity enabled AUPHA to establish an Office of Educational Opportunity to develop and administer programs to increase minority representation in the field of health administration.[14] Since then, 1,372 students have already participated in 10 annual summer health administration internship programs across the United States in over 184 hospitals, neighborhood family care centers, family clinics, and health associations. Of the students, 74 percent were Black, 7 percent Asian American, 10 percent Hispanic, 2 percent Native American, and 6 percent members of other minority groups. Their preceptors recommended 86 percent of them for the profession of health administration.

Kellogg Foundation

Since 1970, the W.K. Kellogg Foundation has been a primary source of support for AUPHA's programs to increase representation in health administration. The Kellogg Foundation played a leading role in developing both the National Work-Study Recruitment Program in Health Administration for Minority Group Students and the National Hospital and Health Services Administration Scholarship and Loan Fund for Minority Group Students. Kellogg continues to support these two programs.

The Commission of Education for Health Administration, with support from the W.K. Kellogg Foundation made the following recommendations: (1) promoting equality of educational opportunity by diminishing barriers related to age, race, and sex, (2) strengthening efforts to recruit women and representatives of all minority groups, (3) maintaining support for existing projects such as summer Work-Study Programs, and (4) arranging special financial support programs for low income students through both public and private agencies.[15]

In 1975, the American Hospital Association, the W.K. Kellogg Foundation, and the Robert Wood Johnson Foundation jointly provided funding to continue the activities of AUPHA's Office of Educational Opportunity over a three-year period.

As a result of this support, the Summer Work-Study Program has been extended from two to a high of 26 cities over the past 10 years. The Scholarship and Loan Fund currently provides financial assistance to more than 112 graduate students in AUPHA graduate member programs.

Other Sources of Funding

State and local health associations, foundations, government agencies, NAHSE, and over 200 hospitals and health facilities have provided advice and funding to the Work-Study program.

Other organizations instrumental in the development and success of AUPHA minority programs include the following: The Blue Cross Plans of Massachusetts, Michigan, and Pennsylvania; the Commonwealth Fund; Manpower Development Program; Health Services Research Foundation of Northern California; the Kaiser Foundation; Linen Systems for Hospitals; Newark and New York–Model Cities; New York City Health and Hospital Corporation; New York State Mental Health Department; Tulane University; United Hospital Fund; Ernest and Mary Weir Foundation; and the Wielbolt Foundation. In addition, the Veterans Administration has had summer intern placements in each city participating in the Work-Study Program.

The Committee on Minority Group Affairs (CMGA) under the chairmanship of Howard W. Houser, Ph.D., of the University of Alabama determines the policies of the Office of Educational Opportunity. This Committee draws its membership from a broad base of health administration and health service organizations. Representatives on the Committee are: Roger L. Amidon, Ph.D., Professor and Chairman, Department of Health Administration, Oklahoma University Health Sciences Center; Felton Armstrong, Director of Management and Analysis, Federal Drug Administration; Barbara Arrington, Admissions Coordinator, Department of Hospital and Health Care, Center for Health Services Education and Research, Saint Louis University; Edna Braddock, Internship Coordinator, Atlanta Urban Corps, Georgia State University; Will Coleman, Administrative Assistant, Health Administration Manpower Division of Membership, American College of Hospital Administrators; Gordon Derzon, Superintendent of Hospitals, University of Wisconsin; Bettejane Kirkpatrick, Assistant to Dean, School of Public Health and Community Medicine, University of Washington; Richard Lichtenstein, Professor, Department of Medical Care Organization, University of Michigan; Frank Mele, Associate Director, Peninsula Hospital, Burlingame, California; Haynes Rice, Executive Director, Howard University Hospital; Raymond Rodgers, F.A.C.H.A., Service Unit Director, USPHS Indian Hospital, Albuquerque, NM; and Hilmon Sorey, Associate Director, Northwestern University, Kellogg Graduate School of Management.

Scholarship aid for education in health administration is administered in a decentralized manner. The local university processes applications. Persons planning to apply to graduate school are well advised to apply early for scholarship aid.

Participants and Graduates

Approximately 1,400 undergraduate students have participated in the National Work-Study Recruitment Program in Health Administration for Minority Group Students. Alumni of the Work-Study Program are becoming increasingly visible in the field. The American Hospital Association has supported the work-study effort.

About 100 students have either obtained graduate degrees in Health Administration or are currently enrolled in AUPHA graduate member programs. Another 100 have pursued graduate level education in business and public administration, medicine, dentistry, and law.

Scholarships and Loans

The W.K. Kellogg Foundation awarded $150,000 for a three-year period (1971–1974) for the development of the National Hospital and Health Service Administration Scholarship and Loan Fund for Minority Group Students. In 1975, the Robert Wood Johnson Foundation joined the W.K. Kellogg Foundation in supporting the fund through 1978.[16] To date, 358 minority students attending AUPHA graduate member programs have been awarded over $435,573 in scholarships or loans distributed through the AUPHA Office of Educational Opportunity.

Other organizations have instituted programs to advance minority educational opportunities in health administration. In 1975, the American College of Hospital Administrators established the Albert W. Dent Work-Study Fellowship as a tribute to Dr. Dent, President Emeritus of Dillard University and the first Black administrator in the professional society. The Dent Fellowship has enabled a minority student to gain additional experience in the health administration field through an eleven-week internship with the American College of Hospital Administrators. The program carries a stipend of $3,000. Qualifying are past Work-Study students enrolled in an undergraduate or graduate program in health service administration.[17]

The American College of Hospital Administrators supports a Foster G. McGaw Scholarship and Loan Fund of $4,000 per year. This fund is administered by the National Association of Health Services Executives, 551 Fifth Avenue, New York, New York 10017. The fund has been used for emergency purposes, and the average award is $600.00.

Traineeships

In 1976, Howard University and Columbia University received special traineeship grants for Health Services Administration from the Bureau of Health Manpower under Section 312B of the Public Health Service Act. This Section authorizes the award of grants to provide support for students who are pursuing training in areas for which there is an unusually high priority need for trained professional manpower.[18]

Work-Study Graduate Program

In 1972, the Office of Health Resources Opportunity entered into a contract with the National Association of Neighborhood Health Centers, Inc., to develop programs to train middle managers already working in community-based health care delivery systems. The program provided mid-level management personnel with the opportunity to attend graduate school without having to give up their jobs. The programs led to an M.P.H. from the University of Michigan and an M.P.A. from the University of Southern California School of Public Administration.[19] Of the 64 minority people who participated, 19 minority people completed the University of Michigan program, and 13 the University of Southern California program.

Since the inception of all these programs, minority student enrollment in AUPHA graduate programs *in toto* has increased from 2 percent (14 of 799) in 1967, to 8.8 percent (187 of 2,106) in 1974, to 12 percent (325 of 2,733) in 1975, to 13 percent (365 of 2,877) in 1976.

The Office of Educational Opportunity of AUPHA attributes the recent plateauing of minority student enrollment to cutbacks in financial aid for graduate programs in health administration, and to the controversy surrounding preferential admission policies for minority students.[20]

In an unpublished study, Kenneth Hill noted that many minority students also attend programs other than those accredited by the Accrediting Commission on Education for Health Services Administration and the American Public Health Association.

Musical Chair Senior Minority Careers

More and more new minority graduates are moving into entry-level jobs. But valid optimism about this happy development must be tempered with a knowledge of the realities of the politics of racism. Black and Puerto Rican health administrators who are demonstrably successful exhibit the musical chair phenomenon. A cycle of job mobility characterizes such senior minority administrators; the Black administrator of Harlem

Hospital replaces the administrator of Detroit General Hospital, who now returns to a Neighborhood Family Care Center. Four years later, he leaves the Neighborhood Family Care Center to replace the Administrator of Charity Hospital, New Orleans, who himself now takes over the original Harlem Hospital job. But with each year, fewer minority hospitals remain to which such administrators can move. Integration has eliminated many Black owned and operated health care facilities. In a report prepared for the National Association of Health Services Executives and published in *Modern Hospitals*, Nathaniel Wesley, Assistant Executive Director, D.C. Hospital Corporation, pointed out that once there were as many as 124 hospitals in the United States catering exclusively to Black patients, 13 of them governmental, and 112 nongovernmental. Today there are but 56, 18 governmental and 38 nongovernmental. The combined income of 34 of these facilities compares favorably with that of the top sales of the four top Black businesses in the country.

Brief Autobiography of a Black Health Administrator

My 22-year career thus far has included service in Black hospitals, in a metropolitan public health department, and in a system of public municipal hospitals, all designed to deliver health services to the poor. At present, improvement of career opportunities for the senior minority administrator continues to lag. I have already commented on the game of musical chairs. The situation is more promising for entry level positions for the young talented minority administrator.

I was admitted to the University of Chicago's graduate program in health administration, having previously been rejected after scoring too low on the entrance examinations. Despite this inauspicious beginning, I subsequently completed the program as the outstanding student in a class of fifteen that also included one Jewish student, one student from India, a physician from Afghanistan, and two women. In its entire 43-year history, the University of Chicago's Graduate Program in Health Administration has graduated but ten Blacks.

One's preceptor is the most important person in one's career development. Everette V. Fox, now administrator of New York University Hospital, throughout the years has been my guide and my role model. I was fortunate to be under his wing. His perseverance in transcending a vicious system during the 1950s inspired me. But what did this same system have in store for me who lacked Everette Fox's ability to get things off his chest in a restrained, dignified manner? In Florida I was exposed to a disgruntled board member who once said to me, "Boy, you ain't no better than that last Nigger we ran away from here." The remark verbalized his annoyance with my temerity in recommending a 5 percent increase for some Black workers who had received no pay raise for three years while other state employees had received a 15 percent wage increase. A final note: the Black workers ultimately received their raise, and the unhappy board member resigned from the board of trustees.

Three of the hospitals in which I once worked are now closed: Kate Bitting Reynolds, Winston-Salem, North Carolina; Florida A & M University Hospital, Tallahassee, Florida; and Jubilee Hospital, Henderson, North Carolina. While they existed, all were indispensable, and their level of patient care compared well with that offered in the larger community. The fate of one of these hospitals calls for special comment. The Kate Bitting Reynolds Hospital closed because the Black community was not organized and failed to grasp the significance and potential of having its own 250-bed health care facility. All employees of this Black hospital were downgraded in rank and responsibility in the process of becoming integrated into the White hospital. The Norfolk, Virginia, Community Hospital survived during the same period, at least in part because of vigorous community involvement. This facility is modern and efficient and enjoys a splendid cooperative relationship with local government.

My decision to move from Norfolk, Virginia, to New York City, the Big Apple, was a hard one. But there was no denying that New York City provided broader opportunities through which I could advance my career in health administration and expand my activities in recruiting minority people for the field. New York City would be an excellent place to start the National Work-Study Recruitment Program, as I was advised by Harold Metcalf, an old friend and formerly Dean of Students, University of Chicago, School of Business. In New York City, I rose from Assistant Commissioner, Office of the Commissioner of Hospitals, to Executive Assistant to the President of the New York City Health and Hospital Corporation that managed all nineteen of the City's municipal hospitals. In the process I had to cram on-the-job training in order to master the politics of health administration in the minority community. I learned how to survive politically. Although I did not receive the Harlem Hospital Directorship that I sought, I was subsequently asked to serve as Acting Director of Harlem Hospital while a permanent Director was being selected. Until the search was completed, I worked with the medical board, the community board employees, the house staff, and the other hospital constituencies. Finally, in New York City in 1974, I became the City's Deputy Health Commissioner under Dr. Lowell E. Bellin, then the City's Health Commissioner and Acting Health Service Administrator. I acted as his liaison and representative to the Health and Hospitals Corporation, to the Comprehensive Health Planning Agency, and to the Health and Hospitals Planning Council of Southern New York. In these roles I helped bring about decisions that would influence the quality and distribution of health care for the citizens of New York City for the next quarter of a century. I claim orchids for the policy direction of the New York City Health Systems Agency. In fairness I must also claim onions for my lesser ability to prevent or resolve the conflict between Dr. Bellin and Dr. John L.S. Holloman, then President of the New York City Health and Hospitals Corporation. Both men were devoted to the betterment of health care. Regrettably, one day a certain letter was written without counsel and the war began. Poor people of New York City would have benefited had these two personalities worked out their ideological differences more successfully.

In 1976, I relocated to Howard University Hospital where I now assist in developing one of the nation's finest medical institutions for patient care, education, research, and prevention of illness.

Final Charge

To the prospective student—and to the minority student—I affirm that the health administrator has an indispensable social role in helping to prolong life and alleviate misery. Early in NAHSE we developed the credo, "One good man and/or woman can make the difference." The principle is still true. The "good" in the credo becomes more important as fallout from the *Bakke* case and from adverse economic factors adds to the troubles minority students encounter in launching a career. Nevertheless, I continue to insist that excellent people with Soul can and will make the difference in all fields, and will make the difference particularly in health administration.

NOTES

[1] Maureen Alth, "The Perils of Pryor." *Newsweek,* October 3, 1977. pp. 60-63.

[2] Charles L. Saunders, "Career Pattern and Mobility Among Blacks in Health Administration." Unpublished memo, August 6, 1977.

[3] Haynes Rice, "To Cure Racism." *Hospitals* 23 (May 1, 1977): pp. 54-56.

[4] Donald Watson, "Minorities and Health Care Administration." *Urban Health* 6, August 1977, p. 29.

[5] Clay E. Simpson, "Opportunities for Minorities in Health Care." *Resume.* National Association of Health Services Executives. Winter 1973.

[6] Haynes Rice, *op. cit.* (note 3), pp. 55–66.

[7]Abraham Flexner, "The Medical Education of the Negro," *Medical Education in the United States and Canada*. New York: The Carnegie Foundation for the Advancement of Teaching, 1910.

[8]*Ibid.*

[9]Donald Watson, *op. cit.* (note 4), p. 36.

[10]*Ibid.*, p. 36.

[11]*Ibid.*, p. 29.

[12]*Ibid.*, p. 34.

[13]Lynette Cooper, *Commentary*, Washington, D.C.: Office of Educational Opportunity, AUPHA, Spring 1977. p. 2.

[14]Clay E. Simpson, Luncheon Address, AUPHA—NAHSE, Washington, D.C., Work-Study Program, August 10, 1977. p. 5.

[15]James P. Dixon, *The Report on the Commission on Education for Health Administration*, vol. 1. Ann Arbor: Health Administration Press, 1975. p. 79.

[16]Lynette Cooper, *op. cit.* (note 13), p. 3.

[17]Albert W. Dent Research Award, National Association of Health Services Executives Pamphlet, New York.

[18]Clay E. Simpson, *op. cit.* (note 14), pp. 1, 3, 4.

[19]*Ibid.*, p. 4.

[20]Lynette Cooper, *op. cit.* (note 13), p. 2.

APPENDIX

I have seized the chance to add an appendix to this paper that contains selected, self-explanatory tables as well as historic highlights excerpted and adapted from a collection compiled by Nathaniel Wesley, Jr., Associate Executive Director, D.C. Hospital Association.

The material in the appendix not only indicates how far the profession of health administration has come but also testifies how far it has yet to go in order to tap the tragically underutilized talents of minority persons.

ANALYSIS OF ALL STUDENTS IN HEALTH ADMINISTRATION
1976-1977

Total Applicants to Schools of Health Administration		Howard	Meharry
Graduate Schools	9,300	48	27
Undergraduate School	1,000	NA	65

Total Students Entering Schools of Health Administration			
Graduate Schools	2,325	15	7
Undergraduate Schools	770	NA	38

Total Students Graduated from Schools of Health Administration			
Graduate Schools	1,800	7	0
Undergraduate Schools	400	NA	32

Adapted from Donald Watson, "Minorities in Health Care Administration." *Urban Health* 6, no. 5 (August 1977): p. 29. Reprinted with permission.

PERCENTAGE OF GRADUATING CLASS
CONSTITUTING MINORITY STUDENTS
AWARDED MASTER'S DEGREES
IN AUPHA-ACCREDITED PROGRAMS 1975

100%–50%		5%–9%	
Howard	100%	U. of Alabama	4%
		Army-Baylor	3%
20%-49%		U. of Chicago	5%
Berkeley	36%	Columbia	4%
UCLA	30%	Duke	3%
U. of Cincinnati	30%	George Washington	5%
U. of Colorado	20%	Georgia State	6%
U. of Mississippi	22%	U. of Minnesota	7%
SUNY	35%	U. of Missouri	6%
		CUNY	7%
10%-19%		Northwestern	7%
Cornell	12%	St. Louis	4%
Florida Int'l	13%	Temple	5%
U. of Michigan	19%	Trinity	2%
U. of Penn	12%	Va. Commwlth U./Med. Coll. Va.	3%
U. of Pittsburgh	13%	Wagner	8%
Tulane	12%	Washington U., St. Louis	6%
U. of Washington	13%	Xavier	6%
		Yale	5%

Source: 1975 Report of AUPHA Office of Educational Opportunity.

MINORITY/NON-MINORITY PERCENTAGE
OF STUDENTS AWARDED MASTER'S DEGREE
AT AUPHA-ACCREDITED SCHOOLS 1975

	Total	% Total
Minority Students	98	9.1%
Non-Minority Students	988	90.9%
Total	1086	100%

WORK-STUDY/NON-WORK-STUDY PERCENTAGE
OF 98 MINORITY STUDENTS AWARDED MASTER'S DEGREE
AT AUPHA-ACCREDITED SCHOOLS 1975

	Total	% Total
Non-Work-Study Students	87	88.8%
Work-Study Students	11	11.2%
Total	98	100%

ETHNICITY AND SEX OF 98 MINORITY STUDENTS
AWARDED MASTER'S DEGREE
AT AUPHA-ACCREDITED SCHOOLS 1975

	Total	%Total	Male	Female	% Male	% Female
Black	73	74.5%	39	34	53%	47%
Asian American	6	6.1%	3	3	50%	50%
Spanish Surname	17	17.3%	14	13	82%	18%
Native American	2	2.1%	1	1	50%	50%
Total/Averages	98	99%	57	51	58%	42%

Source: 1975 Report of AUPHA Office of Educational Opportunity.

HISTORIC HIGHLIGHTS OF BLACK HOSPITALS IN AMERICA

prepared by Nathaniel Wesley, Jr.
Associate Executive Director
D.C. Hospital Association
Washington, D.C.

The old Freedmen's Hospital (1863) is the oldest United States institution devoted to the patient care and professional training of Black people.

The first institution for the exclusive care of indigent colored people was organized in the city of Augusta, Georgia, immediately after the Civil War by an assemblage of colored men.

The first recognized Black hospital in America was Provident Hospital in Chicago. It was founded in 1891 by Mr. Daniel Hale Williams.

The second Black hospital to be established in America was the Frederick Douglas Hospital in Philadelphia. It was founded in 1895 by Dr. Nathan Francis Mossell.

The exclusion of Black physicians from the medical staffs of White hospitals is the major reason that small Black hospitals were founded over the years by Black physicians and others.

Slater Hospital, Winston-Salem, North Carolina, was founded in 1901, by R. J. Reynolds so that sick Black employees of the tobacco company could seek medical care. The hospital closed between 1919 and 1921.

The National Hospital Association was organized in 1923 as a constituent member of the National Medical Association. The purpose of the society was to bring to bear all the forces possible in controlling the unfavorable conditions existing in Negro hospitals. The National Association of Health Services Executives (NAHSE) was organized in 1968 to continue the struggle for better hospital services for the poor and disadvantaged.

During the period of hospital segregation that excluded Black physicians from training at White hospitals and medical centers, Freedmen's Hospital, Washington, D.C., and George W. Hubbard Hospital, Nashville, Tennessee, served as training sites for the overwhelming majority of Black physicians. These institutions are national monuments to Black medical education.
Both now have new, modern expanded hospital facilities.

The 1938 Directory of Negro Hospitals in the United States (published by the National Hospital Association) indicates the following: 105 Negro Hospitals, 30 Approved by the American College of Surgeons, 3 Affiliated with White Hospitals.

Kate Bitting Reynolds Memorial Hospital, Winston-Salem, North Carolina, was completed in 1938, with donations from the community, including $125,000 from the Brown and Williamson Tobacco Company. The hospital was built as a protest against Black physicians losing patients to White hospitals.

In 1938, fourteen Negro hospitals provided internships for Black physicians. These included: John Andrews Hospital, Tuskegee, Alabama; Freedmen's Hospital, Washington, D.C.; Brewster Hospital, Jacksonville, Florida; Provident Hospital, Chicago, Illinois; Homer Phillips Hospital, St. Louis, Missouri; St. Mary's Hospital, Missouri; Lincoln Hospital, Durham, North Carolina; L. R. Memorial Hospital, Greensboro, North Carolina; Flint Goodrich Hospital, New Orleans, Louisiana; Provident Hospital, Baltimore, Maryland; General Hospital #2, Kansas City, Kansas; St. Agnes Hospital, Raleigh, North Carolina; Mercy Douglas Hospital, Philadelphia, Pennsylvania; and George Hubbard Hospital, Nashville, Tennessee.

In 1946, there were fewer than 1,000 hospital beds to care for 1,000,000 Black people in Mississippi.

Sydenham Hospital in New York City was considered by many in 1948 to be the nation's pioneer hospital in medical staff integration.

From 1932 to 1950 the Federal Security Agency of the Public Health Service sponsored National Negro Health Week programs throughout the country. As part of the National Negro Movement, the annual week long program of health events emphasized the need for better health status of the Negro people.

In 1945, the National Medical Association strongly advocated, under the leadership of Dr. Emory I. Robinson, the integration of the Veterans Administration hospital system. In 1954, the VA system ordered the end of segregation of all its hospitals.

A survey of hospital discrimination in southern California (including Los Angeles) revealed that of 4,815 attending physicians on hospital staffs, only 32 were Black.

"The lack of adequate hospital facilities is perhaps the greatest single deterrent to the acquisition of adequate medical care by the Negro. The lack is keenly felt both by the patient and doctor."

Dr. John E. Moreley, Director
Cancer Prevention Center
Sydenham Hospital, 1949

A 1956 Chicago Urgan League survey of Negro appointments to White hospitals revealed that only 16 of Chicago's 226 Negro physicians were on medical staffs of predominantly White hospitals.

As of 1956, there were no Negro physicians serving on the staff of predominantly White hospitals in Atlanta, Nashville, or New Orleans.

From 1948 to 1961, southern states received a large proportion of the $1,600,000,000, which the federal government provided for hospital construction. Of 90 hospitals built in Georgia during this period, 83 were constructed with Hill-Burton money and were segregated facilities.

It took Drs. Hubert A. Eaton, Daniel D. Roane, and S. James Gray almost ten years (1954–63) of litigation and court battles to win the right to staff privileges at James Walker Memorial Hospital of Wilmington, North Carolina. Community Hospital, the Black hospital in Wilmington, served Black patients only and had a biracial staff.

The Imhotep National Conference on Hospital Integration was conceived and organized by Dr. W. Montague Cobb in 1956. Imhotep means "He who cometh in peace." The conference brought together all persons interested in the problems of hospital services for Black patients and privileges for Black physicians. The organization's purpose was "the elimination of segregation in the field of hospitalization and health." The conference met from 1957 to 1961.

During the period 1953 to 1963, fifteen Black schools of nursing closed.

"The Negro hospital is dead. The Civil Rights Act killed it."

Hiram Sibley, Executive Director
Hospital Planning Council of
Metropolitan Chicago
November, 1967

"Inherent in the situation [plight of Negro hospitals] is the feeling on the part of Negroes involved that the product of their sweat and toil over the years will be taken away in the name of progress and that they will find themselves again at the bottom of the ladder where they started."

Dr. W. Montague Cobb
Editor, *Journal of the
National Medical Association*
May, 1976

GENERAL SUMMARY
NONPROFIT COMMUNITY HOSPITALS

Total Number of Hospitals   34
    Private Community   29
    Church Supported   5

Total Number of Beds	4412	Total Payroll $91,909,000[1]
Total Operating Expenses	$170,816,300[1]	Total Employees 10,242[1]

COMPARISONS WITH TOP 100 BLACK BUSINESSES[2]

	Black Community Hospitals	Top 100 (1976)
Total Employees	10,242	5,639

Total Sales of Top Four Companies in Top 100

Company	1976 Sales
Motown Industries	$50,000,000
Johnson Publishing	47,600,000
Johnson Products	43,500,000
Fedco Foods	37,000,000
Total Sales	$178,100,000

Total Operating Expenses of 34 Black Community Hospitals

$170,816,300

[1]*Five of the 34 listed community hospitals did not report operating data to AHA for 1975. The average data for each category as reported above was used to derive the report figures.*

[2]*This comparison is for informational purposes only. As nonprofit institutions, most hospitals are reimbursed on a cost plus formula. The total operating expenses should approximate the level of expected hospital revenue.*

The Curious Hybrid
13   The Physician-Health Administrator

Lowell Eliezer Bellin, M.D., M.P.H.

Today, fewer physicians become health administrators than in the past. Those who continue to do so provide an indispensable leaven to the field. Physicians do not lightly abandon the influence and prestige of the clinic in order to embrace a profession subject to the suspicion, if not the denigration, of clinicians and colleagues who tend to view them as adversaries. What, then, attracts and retains those physicians who choose to join the field? This chapter has application, of course, not only to the physicians but to the dentists, pharmacists, optometrists, and podiatrists who become health administrators each year, and there are insights here that relate to nonclinicians as well.

Lowell Eliezer Bellin has been an internist and health administrator, and is former Health Commissioner of Springfield, Massachusetts, and of New York City. (L.E.B.)

Introduction

There is no alternative. The statistics do not allow it. There simply are not enough physicians to go around who, by formal training or experience, are or want to be health administrators. Most posts in health administration, therefore, are filled and will continue to be filled by non-M.D.s.

A census of students in master's degree programs in health administration would verify that physicians constitute a minority of the enrollment in graduate schools of public health, business administration, or public administration. Moreover, physicians now so enrolled or ever so enrolled constitute but a tiny minority of all licensed physicians in the country. And even fewer health administrators already possessing the master's degree ever go on to medical school.

How then are these relatively few M.D.-health administrators used? What can be the unique contribution of this hybrid?

The Worth of the Physician as Health Administrator

The top brass in the public health departments of the states and larger cities who rank from bureau director through assistant commissioner, associate commissioner, deputy commissioner, and commissioner, are generally M.D.-M.P.H.s. The most common combination of degrees held by the M.D.-health administrator is that of the Doctor of Medicine and Master of Public Health. Similarly, the executive directors of some of the most prestigious medical center complexes known for tertiary care, clinical research, and medical education are M.D.-health administrators with or without the M.P.H.

Most M.D.s and M.D.-M.P.H.s work in those administrative posts that call particularly for the physician's firsthand, technically detailed knowledge to formulate and

---

Lowell Eliezer Bellin, M.D., M.P.H., is Professor of Public Health at Columbia University's School of Public Health, and former Commissioner of Health for New York City.

implement wise clinical policies. It is a physician who most often heads up the hospital outpatient department or oversees the clinical services of the proprietary or voluntary nursing home. In a health department, a physician customarily directs communicable disease or chronic disease epidemiology, maternal and child health services, prison health services, or health care quality control activities.

To be sure, the physician who is a full-time clinical practitioner may look askance at the physician who is a full-time health administrator. Yet, practicing physicians, who are restive at best under any managerial controls, presumably are more likely to be cooperative when a physician rather than a nonphysician is calling the administrative shots in their work habitat. Although the practitioner may habitually scorn the physician administrator as something of a traitor to his or her professional class, the practitioner will concede a similarity of educational and experiential background, albeit temporally remote, on the grounds that (1) the physician-administrator and the practitioner took identical courses in medical school, and (2) the physician-administrator, like the practitioner, once took care of actual patients. Thus, there may be a helpful sense of authentic collegiality, of shared *angst* and insights, that is often lacking in the functional confrontation between the nonphysician health administrator and the clinical practitioner.

In Africa and South America some ambitious individuals obtain medical degrees with no intention of pursuing a traditional medical career for very long. Rather, they plan to use the medical degrees as a bona fide symbol of intellect, as a badge of academic honor, as a culturally sanctioned leverage useful for a career in politics. The medical degree is a ticket to governorship of a province or even to the position of prime minister, not just minister of health. In the United States the law degree sometimes serves this purpose.

The medical degree connotes enormous prestige in the United States as well. As attitudinal surveys have shown, the status of the physician in American society is second only to that of a Justice in the Supreme Court. For this reason alone, if for no other, the possession of the medical degree confers undeniable advantages upon the M.D.-health administrator.

But, of course, it is more than prestige. As previously mentioned, M.D.-health administrators can apply their relevant medical knowledge and skills to the practice of health administration. They have worked in hospitals as physicians. They bring to graduate school and to their careers in health administration a wealth of personal experience that can enrich their professional performance in their new vocation.

These observations are not intended to imply that the medical degree alone ensures that physicians will become better health administrators than their graduate school classmates who have no previous medical background. Certainly, no statistical correlation exists between clinical skills and administrative performance.

However, the contrary absolutist claim is equally incorrect, specifically (1) that physicians are genetically deficient as potential health administrators, or (2) that the characteristic medical school education of physicians has imposed upon them a trained incapacity ever to become competent health administrators. In the controversy that has smouldered over the years between the proponents for M.D.-health administrators versus proponents for non-M.D.-health administrators, hyperbole has sometimes supplanted common sense. It has been alleged, for example, that the clinical knowledge the physician possesses is superfluous to the needs of the health administrator. However, sagacious non-M.D.-health administrators in fact make it a policy to acquire clinical knowledge themselves, to educate themselves in those aspects of clinical medicine particularly relevant to health administration. Health administration is more than keeping the sheets clean, the food hot, the workers content, the professionals quiet, and the clientele happy. Superior health administrators do not sequester themselves intellectually from the technical concerns relating to the care and treatment of patients.

Let us turn now to the practicing physician in his or her pure state before the hybridization of health administration sets in.

Contentment of the Practicing Physician

The practicing physician enjoys satisfactions. They are manifest in the portrayal of therapeutic heroes of novels, cinema, and television reruns. The patient is a supplicant in distress. His or her physiologic and emotional helplessness is to be mitigated by the white-gowned, stethascoped professional. Names of fictional physicians writ large have become household words, more promptly recognized by the layperson than the names of Drs. Osler, Mayo, and Meninger.

Ingenuity exercised on behalf of the dangerously ill patient has always been the stuff of drama. The practicing physician, whether fictional or real, is a combination of knight-errant, wizard, secular priest, and more. By applying scientific knowledge, psychological insight, and technical skills, by intervening directly in order to ease pain, prolong life, or bring a child into the world, the physician imitates the very Creator.

Nor are the gratifications of medical practice limited to the intangible. No other learned professional is more likely to be as generously rewarded with the sweet life. The practicing physician partakes of the best of the spiritual and the physical worlds, from helping humankind in the most indispensable biological way, and from prospering in a gratifying personal materialistic way. The consequent prestige awarded the physician for esoteric knowledge, for service, and for affluence is formidable.

Evolution of Physician into Health Administrator

Why, then, do some physicians, already or potentially clinical practitioners, become public health professionals? Why exchange the operative idealism of practice for the less evident joys of health administration? Why exchange application of diagnostic and therapeutic skills for immersion in the paperwork and intrigues of health administration? What seductive pull can bring about so unusual a switch in the career of an otherwise typical physician? What evolution of thinking causes some physicians to abandon the independence of fee-for-service clinical practice to take up a salaried box in an organizational chart?

After all, the majority of physicians who now occupy full-time positions in public health never intended to claw their way through the competitive years of premedical college and medical school for the purpose of becoming some day comprehensive health planners, executives of hospitals, experts in health care quality and cost control, specialists in medical manpower, savants in third-party reimbursement, or seers in health insurance. Most physicians holding such jobs are retreads who once too participated in the conventional academic lock step leading to clinical practice and maybe even to clinical research and clinical teaching. But somewhere during their career odyssey they felt impelled to veer away—at first tangentially, later at a sharper angle—from the direction of more than 95 percent of their colleagues, to end up playing other professional roles, eventually deemed by these same colleagues to be disparate, marginal, and often hostile to the immediate interests of clinical practitioners.

The Colorless Administrator

A mandatory scene recurs in the war movies. The scene involves dialogue about the dismal fate awaiting the officer who cannot make it in combat, or who has suffered physical or emotional disability. The fate is the despised desk job.

"Please don't put me behind the desk! I don't want to push paper for the rest of my life. Send me back to the fighting—where my men are! I can't take a desk job!" So does the anguished officer plead with his superior in the *de rigueur* scene. One wonders how the United States ever won a war if administrative posts in the military have been reserved exclusively for the inept.

Similarly, the cop on the beat, or in the patrol car—yes, this is the stuff of drama. Similarly, the spy in the furtive service of his government, yes. Even the salesman, yes.

155

Nobility, courage, pathos abound in the field and go with the territory in contrast to the In Box or the water cooler. There is little dramatic heroism to be mined from a central office milieu where all presumably is safety or dullness. The administrative brass are perceived as exchanging memoranda, consuming coffee, and sabotaging the innovations of the real people in the field. The administrator is grey, or at least his caricature is.

There are occasional exceptions. Although a television series about the dilemmas of a mythical mayor was dropped a few years ago for want of viable ratings, a book and the movie made money portraying the professional and emotional trials of a police commissioner. Administration need not always take a back seat like a muted Greek chorus. A spate of Executive Suite novels have dealt with the triumphs and agonies of M.B.A. types in industry. Political novels and plays have been a staple in fiction, providing insights in the public administration of the elected, if not necessarily appointed, officials.

The health administrator is almost invisible. Anyone with predilections toward medicine is likely to be attracted to practice or research, where there is a plethora of role models in popular fiction and in journalism. Under such adverse circumstances, where and why do M.D.-health administrators originate? My own career can serve as a case study of one's evolution from clinician to health administrator.

From Clinic to Office: A Case Study

Pre-Medical School

Like most skeptical premedical students, I did not for long take seriously the earnest protestations of the medical school catalogs about the desirability of liberal arts courses as prerequisites for entering medical school. Certainly I agreed in theory with the principle that a broad liberal arts education was indispensable for the future healer. I simply did not believe that the medical schools abided by this principle in their procedure of sorting out which candidates to admit and which to reject. The medical school catalogs themselves belied their alleged partiality toward an extensive liberal arts education. The premedical courses that were categorized in the catalogs as required (introductory biology, chemistry, and physics, organic chemistry, calculus), plus those premedical courses categorized as desirable or recommended (embryology or comparative anatomy, quantitative analysis, scientific German or French) added up to the curricular program of a premedical major in zoology *cum* minor in chemistry, or vice versa. Furthermore, many premedical students who calculated the odds believed that superior academic performance in the physical sciences was more impressive to medical school admissions committees than an equivalent academic performance in any premedical liberal arts.

So when I applied to the medical schools, my own premedical transcript showed precious little didactic background in the liberal arts. I might as well have gone to college on the moon for all the educative good the nation's foremost scholars in literature, economics, and philosophy on the college faculty did for me. I simply had been unable to fit their courses into a curriculum already jam-packed with lectures and laboratories in the hard sciences. This typical curricular experience of the premedical student—isolated from immersion in the liberal arts—is unlikely to sensitize him or her overly much to the broader social issues relevant to the clinical practice of medicine, let alone those issues relevant to public health. Since the hard science curriculum is practically devoid of such sensitizing experiences, the interested student theoretically might look to extracurricular activities for them. But the typical premedical student has little or no time to devote to extracurricular activities. Premeds are not to be found on the college crew, on the college newspaper, or on the membership rolls of the college's political union—not, that is, if they want to beat out their academic competitors in the scramble toward acceptance by some accredited medical school in the United States. In short, the premedical college experience inside or outside of classes is unlikely to move the would-be future physician toward the direction of public health and health administration.

Medical Schools

Are such interests in public health and health administration inculcated during the four years of medical school? For most fledgling physicians the first curricular contact with health administration takes place in medical school. The student is often less than aware of the encounter. Formal course work in biostatistics and epidemiology often complements the traditional basic sciences of the first and second years at medical school. That the material in these courses constitutes part of the basic science armamentarium of the health administrator even more than it does that of the average practitioner is rarely communicated to the student. To the extent that he or she thinks about it at all, the medical student concludes that these courses apply primarily to the practice of internal medicine, pediatrics, surgery, and obstetrics where morbidity, mortality, and case fatality rates bear review.

Later, the medical student may be exposed to other elements of health administration under the aegis of the variously named Departments of Preventive Medicine, Community Medicine, Family Medicine, Social Medicine, or Environmental Medicine. The student may be exposed to such subjects as public health law, public health programs, and the politics of public health. In view of the extraordinarily crowded curriculum of medical school, almost never is sufficient time allocated for any readings or lectures beyond the barest introductory level.

Nevertheless, for a small percentage of students each year, even this limited exposure to health administration proves to be critical. For them the courses are an unanticipated revelation. For the first time, medical students can infer that an option to clinical practice or research exists. The more perceptive students come to understand that, without competent and devoted health administrators, little clinical practice or research would exist as we know it. Until they are exposed to these courses, it would ordinarily never occur to students that there is a distinction between, say, internal medicine and health care delivery. Now some begin to realize that there is actually a respectable and voluminous literature associated with the latter as well as with the former. This insight is yet to be grasped by the average physician already in practice.

It is unlikely that at this relatively early stage the medical student will conclusively decide on a career in health administration. Still, a seed has been planted. Even the majority who will go on to clinical practice or research will have a better understanding of the anatomy and physiology of health care delivery than did the medical students of a generation ago. A few enthusiasts among the students may take advantage of additional offerings, if they are available, in courses related to health administration.

When I was a medical student, the curriculum was influenced by the Dean, who was an internist with a deep interest in preventive medicine, public health, and family medicine. In my senior year I spent two compulsory months on a public health clerkship. This included seminars of public health interests and visits to work sites of the New York City Health Department. Specialists in public health explained to us the implications of what they did. We met with the leadership of the Health Insurance Plan of Greater New York (HIP), then viewed by many in organized medicine as dangerously radical for its prepaid capitation method of reimbursement in a multispecialty group practice setting. We medical students spent time as assistants or observers in the offices of private practitioners in family practice. And, best of all, each medical student was assigned a complete family to look after.

My assignment was the family of a longshoreman. This was particularly exhilarating, since the social evils fictionalized in *On The Waterfront* were being investigated at the time. My job was to carry out a comprehensive analysis of the health status of each family member: the father, the mother, the four children. I was to complete an inventory of their health and relevant social needs. I was to identify the nonprofit agencies that could serve as a source of health and social services to address these needs. For two months I stayed glued to this family. I met with the school principal and teachers of the children. I got to know the biological and psychosocial dynamics of this family in a professional depth more profound than any I would ever develop during my subsequent clinical career.

But even at a medical school that unabashedly promoted formal education in public health, that proselytized for a family approach to care when family medicine was still a novel expression, the signals about the proper status of public health were ambiguous and contradictory. (1) We students got the impression that inadequate academic performance in public health on the part of medical students would not have the same serious consequences as, say, inadequate performance in biochemistry or surgery. (2) The public health professionals, either full-time or adjunct faculty, were a diverse lot. To us medical students, a surgeon was a surgeon, and an ophthalmologist, an ophthalmologist. We knew what these clinical specialists purported to do. But, what was an M.D.-public health specialist supposed to do? This seemed less clear. There seemed to be so many kinds of public health specialists and so many different programs. Operationally, from the standpoint of a career as a physician, was the field of public health even definable, with defensible boundaries encompassing a solid body of knowledge? The amorphous inchoate nature of the field made us nervous. (3) The National Board Examination in public health was 90 minutes long. Examinations in all other courses were 180 minutes long. This suggested quantitatively that public health was half as important.

It may have been the luck of the draw, but we encountered few people in public health who could serve as culture heroes for us, performing that indispensible modeling role that certain internists and surgeons, for example, were already in the process of fulfilling for many medical students in the class. No later than the first few months of the senior year, each medical student has to plan seriously for his or her internship. This means at least preliminary consideration of the specialty that the student will enter, since one's residency depends in part on the type and locale of one's internship. The yearning for a culture hero after whom to model oneself is no symptom of arrested adolescence, but part of the procedure of socialization that is an indispensable feature of professional education. Medical students want to become internists, or general surgeons, or family physicians, or gynecologists, or psychiatrists, not only because this or that field demands less or more, or pays better, or has more convenient hours of work but also because the medical student is attracted to the specific field by the charisma of specific clinical specialists on the faculty or hospital staff. In the charismatic competition between clinicians and public health professionals in my senior year, the clinicians won overwhelmingly. Not a single person in the senior year at my medical school, including me, planned at graduation to enter public health as a full-time career.

During the past thirty years, however, medical schools throughout the country have come to place greater emphasis on public health in the curriculum. More medical schools now require all students to study biostatistics and epidemiology. Presentations on the intricacies of Blue Cross and other health insurance increasingly infiltrate the lecture halls of medical schools. Nevertheless, such material in the curriculum still lacks the legitimacy of human anatomy and the Krebs cycle of carbohydrate metabolism. In the medical schools, substantive inequities in the treatment of public health as a teaching discipline persist.

On graduation day I would have ridiculed the notion of my entering public health and health administration as a career. At most, my public health clerkship had represented a pleasant diversion, a two-month period of rest and rehabilitation, an ephemeral escape from the heavy specialties that had occupied my senior year at medical school. Surely I had not endured all those rigors and tensions of my premedical and medical school years to enter a professional career that would address itself organizationally to battling tuberculosis and venereal disease and elevating the immunization level of the populace, socially important as all these activities undeniably were. No, I had survived all this educational trial by ordeal in order to become a real doctor, not a medically degreed administrator and social worker.

Internship and Residency Years

My professional plans? After flirting briefly with the idea of a career in pediatrics (I liked children), thereafter orthopedics (I would make the lame walk), I decided upon radiology as my specialty. Diagnostic puzzles were intriguing. The radiologists on the faculty were competent, sagacious, witty, and consummate men of the world. On the advice of a radiologist I knew, I signed up for a straight internship in internal medicine as a useful preparatory year for the field.

As it turned out, the diagnostic and therapeutic puzzles of internal medicine proved to be even more intriguing to me than radiology. Internists supplanted radiologists as my personal role models. The Veterans Administration Hospital, where I spent my straight internship in internal medicine, was blessed with an extraordinarily talented group of attending internists from the affiliated medical school faculty. I stayed on at the V.A. Hospital for a year as Assistant Resident in Internal Medicine. I had fallen utterly in love with clinical medicine. I looked forward to a career of clinical practice. I was content.

Not only did clinical practice offer positive attraction, but my periodic contacts with the administrators of hospitals were characteristically negative. One incident is worth summarizing in part:

The Hospital Director, the chief executive, was a physician who had once been a full-time clinician and had since become a full-time administrator. Like most house officers, I followed the prudent policy of steering clear of hospital administrators. To clinicians, administrators are objects of indifference at best, and hostile obstacles at worst. One day I was summoned to the office of the Hospital Director to explain the circumstances of my having discharged a certain politically well-connected patient despite his vigorous objections. The patient, a veteran like all other patients, had complained to the local chapter of an important national veterans' organization. The local chapter had seen fit to take up his cause. I had thereby given offense to the veterans' organization whose support it was imprudent to forfeit. The Hospital Director emphasized that he had no intention of being critical. He just wanted to collect the facts in order to respond intelligently to the veterans' organization.

As I heard all this, I felt I had been absolutely correct in discharging a patient who had already received more than his maximal hospital therapeutic benefits and was now needlessly occupying a bed. Maybe the hospital executive could be intimidated by this veterans' organization—but certainly not I, in my unassailable position as underpaid and overworked health officer in a teaching V.A. hospital. I felt priggishly self-righteous. My sympathies for the Hospital Director were miniscule. This former clinician, once a real doctor who had unaccountably abandoned clinical practice for the role of administrator, certainly had no one now but himself to blame. It was his own fault if, for the sake of maintaining the hospital, he was forced to truckle to a variety of people, many of whom were clearly his moral inferiors. Administration is politics, I smugly told myself, and politics is dirty.

In my mind I contrasted, on the one hand, hospital administration, with all its compromise and conciliation, with, on the other hand, clinical practice, with all its striving for diagnostic and therapeutic truth. Yes, clinical practice was clean and worthy of the attentions of the person who would strive to accomplish significant things. I was grateful that I was becoming a healer rather than an administrator and politician.

Air Force

I learned to modify these simplistic views during my two years in uniform. In the Air Force I soon found out that, unless I personally involved myself in health administration, I would become incapable of practicing internal medicine properly.

I was Chief of Internal Medicine at the Air Force Hospital. Four junior physicians reported to me. Early in my Air Force career I noted that our internal medicine services were hobbled by delays in communicating and recording chemistries from the hospital's clinical laboratory. Discussion and protests proved of no avail. I brought my complaint directly to the Colonel who commanded the hospital. He promptly saw to it that orders be cut appointing me Chief of Laboratory Services to supplement my responsibilities as Chief of Internal Medicine. Within a week, work flow from the laboratory improved as a result of my applying judicious attention to certain personnel and procedures. Hospital length of stay declined as laboratory results came back more quickly.

Then another bottleneck that hitherto had been obscured by the laboratory problem manifested itself. Communicating and recording x-ray reports dictated by the Air Force Hospital's weekly visiting civilian radiologist were being delayed. Again I complained to the Colonel, and again I had my administrative duties expanded, now to include those of Chief of Hospital Radiology. Work flow in the x-ray department then improved, and patient length of stay at the Air Force Hospital declined further.

This was the first time in my career as a physician that I had experienced gratification from health administration. Before this incident, I had never realized the degree to which quality and efficiency of health care delivery depend upon the degree of competence of health administration. I understood viscerally that the most superbly performed laboratory tests and the most brilliantly interpreted radiographic studies are little but academic exercises if the information fails to arrive in the clinician's hands in a timely fashion. I began to consider whether these administrative activities—traditionally ignored by medical schools and scorned by complacent clinicians—deserved the clinicians' serious attention. I was becoming more cognizant of the place health administration should appropriately occupy in the ecology of health care.

Civilian Teaching Hospital

Two years of service with the Air Force interrupted my residency in internal medicine. When I returned to civilian life, I continued my residency in a civilian teaching hospital. I briefly considered applying for the chief residency. I was dissuaded. Colleagues pointed out that most chief residencies in internal medicine include numerous administrative responsibilities. "Why waste your time pushing paper when you can be learning something real?" they argued, thereby taking a gratuitous swipe at administration. I paid attention to them. I signed up for a National Institute of Health Fellowship in cardiology, where I could perfect myself in a subspecialty. Thus, my return to the atmosphere of a teaching hospital and medical school center served to neutralize the nascent interests in health administration nurtured by my Air Force experience.

Israel

The pendulum was to swing back once more toward administration a year later. Between July, 1957, and June, 1958, I worked in Israel, the first six months as a teaching fellow in cardiology at the Rothschild Hadassah University Hospital in Jerusalem, and the second six months as Acting Chief of Medicine at the Hayim Yassky Hadassah Negev Hospital in Beersheba. At the time the poor quality of Israel's civilian administration, by British or American standards, if not by Middle Eastern standards, was a well-publicized national scandal. The generally bad quality of this administration in private and public agencies had its representative counterpart in the health administration of the country as well. The Hadassah Hospitals in Jerusalem and Beersheba were administered better than most health facilities and programs in Israel, perhaps because of the cultural influences of American philanthropic benefactors. But one had to be singularly obtuse not to perceive the enervating impact of poor administration of the country's health services upon the quality of delivery of care to the population. The salutary effects of excellent technical quality of care were cancelled out partially by the sloppy administrative management of health services. The operative attitude existed (presumably harking back to socialist ideology) that anyone with common sense and with proper social commitment can be an administrator. Certainly very few people in posts of health administration had ever received formal training in administration.

My six months' experience in Beersheba drew me back to health administration. The burgeoning population of the Negev exerted increasing pressure upon the relatively few internal medicine hospital beds available. New hospitals in Beersheba and Eilat were still in the planning stage. It was necessary to ration hospital bed days among the sickest patients. We developed the unusual policy of discharging patients as soon as they showed positive signs of responding to therapy. We worked closely with public health nurses and the hospital outpatient department in order to hyper-integrate posthospital care with the inpatient care of every person who was hospitalized. Average length of hospital stay in the Department of Internal Medicine in Beersheba declined. In order to deliver maximal effective internal medicine care to the population of the Negev, the only internal medicine department of the only hospital in the Negev was compelled to exercise administrative ingenuity. I found myself immersed in policy questions of hospital admission and discharge, in the dilemmas of applying finite resources. Each administrative decision had life and death implications of enormous statistical importance to the total population.

In Beersheba I relearned my lesson of the United States Air Force: that internal medicine and health care delivery are not precisely the same thing. The subject I had learned in medical school and during my internship and residency had been internal medicine. What I had been forced to teach myself under fire in the trenches had been health care delivery. Health care delivery was a subset of health administration.

Nevertheless, I gave no serious consideration to doing health administration full-time. After a year of service in Israel, I returned to the United States to enter private solo practice as an internist and cardiologist.

Private Practice: Areas of Frustration

After having been in private practice for no more than six months, I found that a paradox was in operation. On the one hand, I was technically overtrained for the bulk of work that one would call traditional internal medicine, much of which was routine. Four years of formal postgraduate training in internal medicine in American hospitals had not prepared me completely for the realities of private practice. Nor had two years of service in the Air Force, or a year of service in Israel. In all my previous work settings, diagnostic and therapeutic problems had first been carefully screened. Only the most interesting would thereafter be served up for my intellectual delectation. The diagnostic and therapeutic problems I had previously encountered in the teaching setting had most assuredly not been anything like the problems that were besetting me as a physician in the private practice of ambulatory care. These new problems seemed to present less intellectual challenge to the sophisticated skills I had been taught. On the other hand, the opposite could also be argued: that, in fact, inhospital education had rendered me technically undertrained for the intellectual demands of ambulatory care. I had received little formal teaching in how to deal with the psychosomatic problems that represented more than 50 percent of my practice. Of what use were my hard-won skills in manipulating electrolytes, for example, if the patient's physiological complaints originated in a less than satisfactory marriage? Once I had eliminated an organic etiology for the patient's chronic fatigue, or abdominal pain, what then? Push tranquilizers? Whatever the explanation for my unhappiness with my daily work, I was patently dissatisfied with what I was doing.

Once I treated a patient for bronchitis. The usual antibiotic and antitussant were effective. Three weeks later, the same patient returned, now in relapse. Again I treated him with the appropriate antibiotic and antitussant. The same sequence of events occurred, first response and subsequent relapse. Was I dealing with a patch of bronchiectasis that was repeatedly reseeding the lungs with infection? I wondered whether bronchography was called for to localize the possible bronchiectasis.

Not necessarily. The patient, who lived in the North End—the Black and Hispanic slum area of the city—suggested a plausible explanation. Heating in his apartment was inadequate, and the landlord allegedly refused to turn up the heat. The environment might be at fault. And so another lesson came home to me. If the patient's explanation was correct, what could I as a practitioner really do? I was not all-powerful. The landlord would be unlikely to listen to me. Should I complain to the City Health Department? Could it be that health administrators on the public payroll would be more effective in preserving the biological health of the patient's lungs than I, a Board-certified internist, with all my application of antibiotics, antitussants, and bacterial culture and antibiotic sensitivity studies?

I had already learned once that internal medicine was not the equivalent of health care delivery. Now I had to conclude that delivery of health care services was not necessarily the equivalent of delivery of health.

During my four years of solo practice as an internist and cardiologist, I tried without success to organize a group practice of internists. My motives were mixed. I wanted to mitigate what had already become a 60- to 70-hour work week. I wanted to increase my income by pooling overhead expenses with other physicians. I wanted to re-evoke the cultural advantages of the collegiality I had missed since leaving the teaching hospitals of my internship and residency training.

Since the immediate prognosis for establishing such a group practice was poor in my city, the alternative that bore consideration was moving from the city and joining a group practice already in existence in another community. Before such a move could be consummated, the city's mayor, who had heard of my plans from a mutual friend, offered me the position of Health Commissioner, with the stipulation that I attend the Harvard School of Public Health on a part-time basis for two years in order to receive my Master's of Public Health degree. The post of City Health Commissioner had been vacant for more than a year. I felt I had little to lose. By taking the job I could temporize and have a chance to rethink my career plans. At worst I would have a few years of practical experience in health administration. Moreover, the possession of an M.P.H. degree would do me no harm, no matter what I would do in the future.

So, in 1962, I formally entered public health on a full-time basis. Other than practicing as camp doctor during summer vacations, I never again performed clinical work.

What Brings Most Physicians into Health Administration?

Proper case studies are supposed to illustrate generalizable principles. Thus far my comments have been partially autobiographical. Why I left a growing private practice in internal medicine and cardiology to become a public health professional should provide insight into some of the reasons for the annual indispensable trickle of family physicians, pediatricians, internists, and occasionally other types of physicians into health administration. Other reasons will be discussed.

Most physicians who ultimately enter a career in health administration do so only after a trial of clinical medicine during their internships, residencies, or even private practice. As already mentioned, sometimes the decision is arrived at because the physician either does not enjoy private practice or is disillusioned with some aspect of practice. Nor need the reasons be altogether negative. The physician may be quite satisfied with private practice, even tolerate its less pleasant elements, but yet be attracted to the broader social canvas that health administration offers.

Unpleasantness of Reimbursement

Most physician practitioners are satisfied with what they are doing. To say this is not to suggest that these physicians are complacent or obtuse for feeling satisfied.

162

Happy is the person who rejoices in his portion. The minority of physicians who are restive are not necessarily more sensitive, more insightful, more compassionate than their colleagues. No hierarchy of operative morality is to be inferred. Some practitioners, on the other hand, are not satisfied.

Fee-for-service, the usual method of reimbursement for practitioners, functions as an incomparable goad toward high productivity, and as an occasional incentive toward overutilization of services, that is, the provision of services justified neither for preventive nor for therapeutic reasons. Whatever else the fee-for-service represents, this method of reimbursement requires the meticulous recording of each fiscally identifiable service to ensure accurate billing. Also necessary are follow-up reminders to pay overdue bills. The physician is obliged to plunge into the business of practice. If the patient does not pay, the physician will deny that patient further care, except in extraordinary circumstances. Some physicians who find this whole process distasteful, yet want to remain clinicians, flee to salaried practice in a group setting or a hospital. Numerous physicians in public health will testify that a contributing cause to their exchange of private practice for public health was their dislike of sending out bills and subsequent dunning letters.

Guilt Over Comfort and Prosperity

Some practitioners find that initially their activities as practitioners satisfy their yearnings to be of service to society. The act of caring for human beings who are humanity's surrogates is spiritually reassuring. They believe that they are applying their skills as optimally as could be expected by at least those social reformers who stop short of demanding heroic materialistic renunciation on the part of physicians and a transfer of the physicians' authority and prestige to the proletariat. Even so, as time goes on, some physicians become uneasy. Something is missing. Sometimes it is hard to take seriously the view that one is serving the poor when one is rich. Of course one remembers the incredibly tough and expensive four-year education in medical school, which was succeeded by another four to five years of internship and residency, and feels some relief. This reassurance of personal self-sacrifice is less readily available today. Although medical school is as tough as ever, some of the anxiety over flunking out has faded. Evidently, the new educational policy is to get as many students as possible through medical school. Once the student is accepted, the chances of academic survival up to the achievement of the medical degree are excellent. The gut-curdling anxiety of medical school of yesteryear is less evident. The four to five postgraduate years of hospital training are hardly years of poverty any longer—not when one can count on salaries ranging from $10,000 to $25,000 per year. Not many apprenticeships in other fields pay anywhere near that well. Thus, existential guilt is now justified. Some public health physicians, not necessarily only the neurotic, account in part for their entering public health as a striving for some sense of dedication and personal self-sacrifice.

Helping Humanity in Large Numbers

Some physicians want to leave their imprint on society. As time goes by, it is no longer enough to intervene on a one-to-one basis on behalf of the individual patient. If the internist has 100 patient visits weekly and works 50 weeks per year, he or she will see 5,000 patients annually. If we assume 4 visits per year on the average per patient, the physician is caring for the biologic and mental well-being of 1,250 separate patients per year. Some physicians ask themselves: "Did I really go through all this to care for only these 5,000 to 10,000 or so patients in my files? Was I destined to be responsible for no more than these human beings?" Put this way, the question can be distressing. The practice becomes somewhat trivial numerically.

At best, the physician can only intervene in behalf of the health of a single patient at a time. He or she has no legal authority over the relevant environment that affects tens of thousands of people. Not so the public health physician who can intervene legally to manipulate the environment on behalf of the health of these tens of thousands. This legal authority inherent in the role of public health physician is what continues to attract and retain some physicians in health administration.

Advantages of Health Administration

The physician who wishes to bring about substantive social change in the distribution, quality, and funding of health services would be wise to keep the following social truism in mind: who controls the means of production of goods and services has much to say about social and economic policy. Government and the hospitals control much of the means of production of health services.

The private citizen is routinely urged every November to vote and thereby participate in the formulation of public decisions. Without such participation, democracy would ultimately wither. One can espouse this view with sincerity. At the same time, it is wise to bear in mind that each private citizen individually has only a trivial statistical impact on any public decision, or, for that matter, on the election of any public official. But the power of the individual citizen is multiplied ten thousand-fold in formulating public decisions at the moment the private citizen assumes an administrative post in the pertinent public bureaucracy.

Similarly, the individual practicing physician is intolerably limited, in terms of what one can do by oneself. In contrast, the health administrator uses staff to get things done. Only the person who has had access to the organization as an instrument to get things done can have insight into the magnificent advantage of the organization over the isolated individual. The insight is hardly subtle. Yet, the advantages of organization come home to the physician when, for the first time, the former M.D.-practitioner, now health administrator, has the occasion to send subordinates on the staff out to do something.

Hitherto the physician in a private office had at the most two or three assistants. Now in an administrative post his or her eyes, ears, and hands have seemed to proliferate and extend to the numerous eating establishments that the sanitarians are inspecting, or to the schools where public health nurses are immunizing, screening, and following up defects in children, or in the legislative body where the legislators are pondering laws that he or she has authorized to be drafted. There is a sense of exhilaration. The public health physician who has tasted such delights finds it hard ever to return to the solitary life. Like the farmer who gets used to the advantage of a mechanical combine, he or she is reluctant to reassume the status of the peasant with a primitive stick with which to scratch the ground.

It is gratifying to play at permanence—to display programmatic semi-immortality. The practicing M.D. cannot do this alone. As part of a collection of physicians who formally share a practice and who abide by ideological policy that he or she has helped to fashion, the physician in group practice can institutionalize himself. However, the physician's striving for semipermanence is more likely to be successful if he or she controls a part or the whole of a health department, a hospital, or some other health enterprise; that is to say, if he or she is unabashedly a health administrator. Certain programs in today's health department continue as the legacies of the health administrators of 30 to 50 years ago. To the professional health administrator this is a source of satisfaction comparable only to the satisfaction received by the architect each time he or she gazes upon a building he or she has designed.

Education

The following only briefly summarizes the health administrator-M.D.'s education. For further details and nuances the reader is advised to consult the American Board of Preventive Medicine. The physician who wishes to become a health administrator usually pursues the following course of study: (1) Medical School: with acquisition of

164

the medical degree (M.D.), four years; (2) Internship: one year; (3) Graduate school of public health with acquisition of Master's of Public Health degree (M.P.H.): one year. The M.P.H. degree for the physician confers formal legitimacy in health administration. (4) Residency in public health preventive medicine: usually two years in a state or city health department or other educational site approved for this purpose by the American Board of Preventive Medicine.

Such a program qualifies the physician to take the examination of the American Board of Preventive Medicine. The candidate who successfully passes the examination becomes a Board-certified specialist in preventive medicine.

There are variations. Some physicians take part or all of their residency training in a clinical specialty, often pediatrics or internal medicine. Thereafter they may take the residency in public health–preventive medicine or go directly to a graduate school of public health for formal education in health administration. Board-qualified and Board-certified pediatricians and internists in particular, some of whom continue in part-time clinical practice, occupy posts in health administration in this country.

14   As Quality Assurance Specialist

Eleanore Rothenberg, Ph.D.

The concept of quality control has belatedly spilled over from manufacturing to human services. The increasing public subsidy of health services has provided this concept with irresistible political impetus. This momentum often meets the sullen resistance of some health practitioners and heads of institutions, who object that outside auditors will henceforth monitor a random sample of the quality of the care they provide. In short, caveat emptor *betokens more and more quality control, particularly when the* emptor *turns out to be the government, or, more precisely, the taxpayer. Whether Professional Standard Review Organizations (PSROs) endure is almost irrelevant, because quality control, and its sometime reluctant partner, cost control, have now become permanent features of health care delivery.*

Eleanore Rothenberg discusses the opportunities in this specialty for the health administrator. (L.E.B.)

Introduction

In 1965, a hospital was held liable for neglecting to assure the quality of care provided by one of its attending physicians to one of its patients, thereby establishing the principle that hospitals (that is, hospital trustees and administrators) are responsible for reviewing patient care and for intervening where such care does not meet professional quality standards.[1]

The now famous *Darling* case involved a young athlete who suffered irreparable damage following the improper application of a cast by one of the hospital's attending physicians. Despite the patient's frequent complaints of severe pain, attention was delayed and his leg had to be amputated.

The patient sued, arguing that the hospital's nurses had a duty to notice the patient's problems and report them to the administrator who, in turn, had a responsibility to alert the medical staff whose duty it was to intervene.[2] The jury concurred, awarding damages, thus establishing a new doctrine of hospital responsibility. This landmark decision has profoundly affected the role of the health administrator as quality assurance specialist.[3]

Two conflicting theories had characterized court decisions until that time. Under the first, the hospital could not be held responsible for the acts of its physicians, who were held to be members of an independent profession "sanctioned by a noble oath, and safeguarded by stringent penalties."[4] The other point of view, according to Somers, held that "...there is the growing evidence that neither oath nor professional penalties are adequate to protect the public against improper medical care...."[5]

By the end of the 1960s, the health profession had accepted the concept that the responsibility for assessing and assuring the quality of medical care falls within the

---

Eleanore Rothenberg, Ph.D., is Executive Director of the New York County Health Service Review Organization.

purview of the health administrator as expressed in the classic work by Avedis Donabedian, *A Guide to Medical Care Administration: Volume II Medical Care Appraisal.*[6] Offered as an administrator's guide, the book identified approaches to medical care appraisal, with administrative action as the objective.[7] In describing his frame of reference, Donabedian states, "The emphasis in this volume is on those methods of appraisal that can monitor, constantly and repeatedly, the quality of care for which a program has assumed responsibility."[8]

The public's demand that medical care be monitored constantly and repeatedly is apparent from the ever increasing federal regulation of care provided and paid out of public funds. Before describing the present role of the administrator in assessing and assuring quality, it may be useful to examine medical care appraisal in historical perspective.

Quality Assurance in Historical Perspective

Most of the literature describing the evolution of medical care assessment sets the beginning as the year 1910, when Abraham Flexner issued his report on medical education.[9] Flexner's survey, which focuses specifically on inadequate medical education in the field of surgery, was the first systematic evaluation of physician performance.

Flexner also identified other problems, such as incompetence, a high rate of unnecessary surgery, fee splitting, and inadequate hospital facilities.[10] These problems were either known or suspected by the existing professional organizations such as the American Medical Association (AMA) and the Association of American Medical Colleges (AAMC). However, it was not until Flexner's recommendations were published that needed reforms were instituted both in medical education and in hospital care.

Between 1912 and 1916, the Clinical Congress of Surgeons, predecessor of the American College of Surgeons (ACS), seeking to develop procedures for the classification and standardization of the nation's hospitals, turned to a Boston physician, Ernest Codman, whose objective methods of evaluating hospital surgical care were then being published.[11]

Codman's methods for abstracting, classifying, and assessing hospital care, on a case-by-case basis, included evaluation of both favorable and unfavorable end results, as well as assignment of "responsibility for the latter [unfavorable results] to errors in diagnostic and technical ability, poor surgical judgment, inadequate care or equipment...."[12] His review methods also incorporated approaches for corrective action, analysis of fatal cases, and a yearly restudy and reevaluation of cases until a condition of stability permitting final judgment has been reached.[13]

In 1916, the ACS, using Codman's method of medical care appraisal based on objective criteria, undertook a survey of chronic appendicitis cases starting with a study of diagnosis, treatment, and outcome, and comparing care in a sample of hospitals of 100 beds or more. The findings were startling. Only 89 of the 692 hospitals studied were able to meet any reasonable standard of quality.[14] According to Lembcke, neither the criteria nor the findings of the survey were ever published, nor were they preserved in the files of the ACS, probably because "the facts elicited by the first survey were so shocking that the survey committee ordered individual survey reports destroyed forthwith."[15]

According to R. Heather Palmer, establishing a national system of outcome evaluation of surgery based on Codman's methods was too threatening to its members, and was rejected by the ACS.[16] Instead, the ACS adopted a program to help define minimum standards for hospitals. These eventually evolved into hospital accreditation requirements and addressed what Donabedian calls structural elements, such as the organization, supervision, and discipline of the medical staff; maintenance of medical records; and hospital governance.

In 1952, the newly created Joint Commission on Accreditation of Hospitals (JCAH) assumed responsibility for hospital accreditation, building on the activities of the ACS between the years 1916 and 1952.[17] Hospitals seeking JCAH accreditation did so on a voluntary basis. Eventually, state hospital licensing laws and Medicare and Medicaid health financing programs incorporated many of the minimal JCAH accreditation requirements.[18]

For the 30 years between the early 1920s and the early 1950s, quality assurance activities thus seemed to be limited to (1) efforts to improve hospital organization, procedures, and facilities; and (2) improvements in the training of physicians through undergraduate and graduate medical education programs.

Lembcke suggests the reasons for this limitation. Reforms in medical education, based on the Flexner recommendations, prevailed because of substantial financial backing to establish new medical schools and improve existing ones. No such financial backing was available for the reform movement concerned with hospital and surgical practice. More important, according to Lembcke, the reforms would have had to be instituted by a professional society of doctors "whose members were directly associated with the hospitals and doctors to be criticized."[19]

Beginning in the late 1940s and early 1950s, the situation began to change. The modern hospital, staffed with well-trained physicians, organized and equipped to deliver more and better medical care services, was becoming the focal point of the health care delivery system.[20] Moreover, new purchasers of hospital care grew up, including private insurers, industry, labor, and government. Hospital admissions were rising rapidly, as were hospital costs. Some believed that a substantial proportion of these hospital admissions were unnecessary.[21] As a consequence, a new element was added to the concept of medical care appraisal, namely, the review or assessment of hospital utilization.[22] Furthermore, the evolution of data handling systems, including the use of computers, made it possible "to process, display, and summarize large masses of data which are relevant to the administrative appraisal and control of utilization and quality."[23]

By 1965, Utilization Review (UR) had become a well-established concept, as evidenced by its inclusion in the 1965 Medicare law.[24] As a condition for participation in the Medicare health care financing program, hospitals and extended care facilities were required to establish standing UR committees and to develop a plan for the review of admissions, lengths of stay, and professional services rendered in the institution. The nongovernmental JCAH, which had developed and applied standards for accreditation of hospitals under private auspices between 1952 and 1965, was given responsibility for certifying hospitals for eligibility to participate and receive payment under the new federal Medicare program.[25] The JCAH accreditation process thus became a quasi-public function and was extended to include evaluation of the hospital's UR plan and committee structure.

One of the most significant contributions to medical care appraisal was the medical audit, developed by Paul Lembcke and his associates.[26] During the late 1940s and 1950s, in one set of studies which employed both process and outcome methods of measuring quality, Lembcke et al. identified wide variations in the rate of surgical procedures (appendectomy) per 1,000 population in selected hospital service areas of New York State.[27] In subsequent studies using explicit criteria and a retrospective case-by-case review method, Lembcke studied the medical necessity of operations on the uterus, ovaries, and fallopian tubes performed at community hospitals as compared with teaching hospitals.[28] The results revealed that, prior to the audit, 80 percent of the operations performed at the teaching hospitals were justified, compared to 29 percent at the community hospitals. After the audit, the percentage of justified operations was comparable in both groups of hospitals (approximately 80 percent). By providing a systematic procedure for feedback, Lembcke's method was effective in reducing unjustified surgical procedures in the community hospital.[29]

Despite these auspicious beginnings, however, medical audit methods were not widely used until recently. Few such studies appeared in the literature until the era

169

beginning around 1960, when a variety of new approaches began to be tested and reported in various parts of the country. In addition to the medical audit approach pioneered by Lembcke, there emerged a new concept known as health accounting, which is a method of sampling cases, based on diagnosis, for in-depth study. The health accounting concept, regarded as a problem-solving approach to the linking of patient care assessment with continuing education of physicians, was first introduced by John W. Williamson in 1967, and was later applied by other researchers.[30]

Despite the seemingly long history and recent burgeoning of research into the methods of medical care appraisal, debates about the state of the art continue. In a recent publication, for example, Robert H. Brook recommended that "...the respective methods (process and/or outcome measures) should be tested as to comparative validity, reliability, and feasibility to determine which is the 'best' approach to use, depending on the purpose of the quality assessment and the [diagnostic] conditions selected for study."[31]

While researchers explore these questions and gather information on methods of measuring and assuring the quality of care, public policy is demanding that methods already known be applied. Various concurrent and retrospective review activities are mandated, for example, under the auspices of the Professional Standards Review Organization (PSRO) program. The JCAH requires that review procedures be conducted by hospitals if they are to maintain their accreditation. The Health Maintenance Organization (HMO) Act of 1973 requires that quality assurance activities be conducted in all federally funded HMOs, and the 1977 Medicare-Medicaid Anti-Fraud and Abuse Amendments to the Social Security Act give high priority to evaluation of care provided in shared health facilities, the so-called Medicaid mills.

With these trends in public policy and the concomitant change in emphasis which has characterized health and hospital administration in recent years, quality assurance has come to be regarded as a growth industry. Brook estimated that approximately 50,000 medical audits or Medical Care Evaluation (MCE) studies concerning the quality of inpatient hospital care would be performed in 1977.[32] This estimate did not include concurrent review functions required under the PSRO program with respect to admissions and continued stays in hospitals, or quality and utilization control programs involving ambulatory and long-term care facilities.

The need for health administrators, researchers, public administrators, and specialists in related disciplines who are interested in this field is, therefore, evident. However, such specialists will need to acquire the necessary education and experience in quality or utilization control if they are to perform effectively their administrative responsibilities for quality assurance programs in medical care settings.

Career Opportunities for Quality Assurance Specialists

Graduates of health administration programs will find opportunities in a variety of federal, state, or local health agencies, in quasipublic agencies such as the JCAH, and in Professional Standards Review Organizations or their successors.

The growth and development of PSROs during the mid-1970s is illustrative. Under Section 1152 of the Social Security Act, the Secretary of the former Department of Health, Education and Welfare (DHEW) [now the Department of Health and Human Services (HHS)] was required to designate 203 PSRO areas, covering the 50 states plus the District of Columbia, Puerto Rico, and various territories (Guam, American Samoa, the Trust Territory of the Pacific Islands).

By the end of 1977, there were at least 185 operating PSROs in the United States, with key staff positions often held by administrators, physicians, and nurses with master's degrees in public health or public administration. Other key staffers included business administration program graduates, registered record administrators, data specialists, and biostatisticians, especially those with a knowledge of utilization review or medical audit functions within hospitals.

170

Many executive directors heading PSROs gained their experience in line or staff hospital administration positions. This writer, for instance, held a senior staff position at an academic medical center as associate director of research and policy analysis before joining the PSRO as deputy executive director (later becoming executive director).

PSROs have had an impact on affected institutions (primarily hospitals thus far) and, therefore, on the demand by these institutions for trained quality assurance specialists. Hospital administrators will, over time, need either to develop an in-house capability in this respect or have it performed by external agencies. State and regional hospital associations, having also developed staff capabilities in this area, are likely to continue this work, since quality assurance programs seem to be here to stay.

In the New York County area, virtually every hospital under the PSRO's jurisdiction viewed delegation of hospital review functions allowed under the federal mandate, as a form of accreditation. Nearly 95 percent requested such delegation. This meant that 35 hospital administrators had to assume responsibility for the quality assurance program mandated under the federal program in order to meet the requirements, including an appropriate and acceptable organizational structure, involving standing committees of the hospital and medical boards; written plans specifying review procedures and policies; commitment of necessary resources, both manpower and material, to assure proper implementation of the review system; and a plan for continuing education and involvement of the medical staff.

The public accountability requirement in the PSRO legislation has also created a demand for such specialists to monitor the monitors of quality care. These supermonitors include the funding authorities and agencies, such as Congress, DHHS (represented by the national and regional offices of the Health Standards and Quality Bureau), fiscal intermediaries for Medicare (Blue Cross and Travelers in New York), agencies for Medicaid (Department of Health and Social Services in New York State), and the federal Medicare Bureau which administers that program in selected hospitals. As a result, quality assurance specialists are surfacing at these agencies, as well as in other federally funded agencies which are required to establish relationships with their area PSROs (for example, Health Systems Agencies and End Stage Renal Disease Program Networks).

Opportunities for quality assurance specialists may also be found in other institutional settings, such as psychiatric and rehabilitation facilities, nursing homes, HMOs, neighborhood health centers, surgicenters, and wherever else health services are delivered and paid for by third-party payers.

Unquestionably, in light of this new emphasis and trend, there will be a need for teachers of such courses and training programs, not only in schools of public health and administration where such course offerings are already on the rise, but also in medical schools, nursing schools, and the rapidly expanding continuing medical education (CME) programs.

At a recent CME conference, discussion among the nation's leading postgraduate medical school educators focused on the desirability of linking performance review to mandatory CME. While there was disagreement among the experts as to whether CME ought to be mandatory and linked to assessment of physician competence, there was no disagreement regarding recent events and their implications for the future. It was noted, for example, that since 1970, a number of states had enacted relicensure laws based on competency, and that a newly created National Commission for Health Certifying Agencies would be examining recredentialing standards and processes.[33]

The quality assurance specialist, therefore, is likely to find new satisfying career opportunities in the area of education.

The Role of the Quality Assurance Specialist

The basic functions of the quality assurance specialist, in almost any setting, will include planning, organizing, staffing, directing, coordinating, and evaluating review activities for which the organization (or division, in the case of the institutional setting) is responsible.

The quality assurance specialist will undoubtedly be called upon continually to identify and interpret statutory requirements which must then be translated into operational programs. The PSRO program provides a good example. The legislation defines the PSRO's primary functions, requiring them to

> Assume responsibility for review of professional activities of institutional providers. PSROs were not required to review non-institutional providers and services under the original law, but could extend their programs to such review, with the approval of the Secretary of DHEW. The 1977 Medicare/Medicaid Anti-Fraud and Abuse Amendments (P.L. 95–142, 42 U.S.C.A. §1320c–4) encourage PSROs to extend review to ambulatory care settings such as out-patient departments and emergency rooms and to shared health facilities, the so-called "Medicaid mills," where they exist in a PSRO area.

> Determine whether (a) services and items are or were medically necessary; (b) the quality of such services meets professionally recognized standards; and (c) services or items provided in hospital or other health care facility could be provided on an outpatient basis or in a less costly facility. In the case of elective admission, the PSRO has the legislative authority to determine (a) and (c) in advance.

> Determine and publish the criteria, by type of care or diagnosis or by other relevant factors, which they use to carry out their mandate.

> Delegate to hospital review committees which can demonstrate their capacity to perform effectively certain review functions required under the PSRO program.

> Maintain and review profiles of patient care and services provided and received, using coding methods to assure confidentiality.

> Utilize the services of practitioners and specialists in carrying out their review responsibilities.

> Apply professionally developed norms of care, diagnosis, and treatment based on typical patterns of practice in the area, including length of stay by age and diagnosis. [34]

In order to achieve such purposes or make them operational, the quality assurance specialist must create or maintain an organizational structure, and must act as the linchpin between the various component parts. In a PSRO this may include developing a functional organization; creating and staffing standing committees of a governing board; and, most importantly, recruiting and training highly motivated and skilled managerial, review, technical, and support staff.

One formidable task for the quality assurance specialist is that of gaining and maintaining physician support for the goals and objectives of the review program as well as their active participation in carrying out the program's mandate. Historically, physicians have resisted efforts to regulate their professional activities, viewing mandated cost and quality control programs as governmental interference with the practice of medicine.

In a recent article in the *New England Journal of Medicine*, David Kessner observed, for example, that "the close professional scrutiny implied by the term 'quality assurance systems' generates apprehension and a sense of alienation in many physicians."[35]

The recent history of the PSRO program and its implementation tends to support Kessner's observation. Since PSRO enactment in 1972, organized medicine has been ambivalent about the PSRO mandate, alternatively seeking to have it repealed, revamped, enjoined, or found unconstitutional. On the other hand, the American Medical Association published, under federal contract, a set of screening criteria to assist PSROs in their review activities. Moreover, many local county medical societies sponsored PSROs that subsequently assumed review responsibilities in designated areas across the country.

In this writer's experience, the attitude among many conservative physicians in the PSRO area was unmistakably hostile. At a meeting of the medical board of one local specialty hospital, for example, where we were to describe the federally mandated peer review system, the feeling was clearly that the PSRO representatives were interlopers.

However, this open and candid opposition was the exception rather than the rule, in part because the founder of the program was a respected and well-known leader in the physician community. During the planning phase, the dean of a large academic medical center, who was also the president-elect of the county medical society, spearheaded the PSRO effort by establishing a committee comprised of physicians representing organized medicine as well as other prominent leaders in the medical community. It was recognized that there would soon be a need for broad representation of the major constituencies within the physician community on the board of directors. Therefore, the first group of physicians to stand for election included individuals of outstanding reputation, representing various specialties, as well as the major hospitals in the area. The politically active committee on interns and residents, the osteopaths, and the local public health agencies specifically were included.

One can conclude, therefore, that the quality assurance specialist will be more likely to enlist and maintain the support of practicing physicians if he or she develops an organization which demonstrates visibly the participation of the local practicing physicians. In hospital settings, this means that the most powerful faculty members or senior attendings should be deeply involved in the program's development and implementation. In an external review agency, such as PSRO, participation by prominent practicing physicians will help (although it will not guarantee) the viability of the review program.

Preparing for a Career in Quality Assurance

To become a specialist in a quality assurance program, the student needs to be armed with knowledge and skills which may be acquired in formal course work alone or in combination with direct experience in a health agency. Most important, perhaps, is experience (line or staff) in a short-term acute care hospital. In recent years, the hospital has become the focal point for community health services and represents the most expensive component in the health care system. Consequently, it is most often the starting point for quality or cost control efforts mandated under publicly funded programs. Moreover, the hospital is the best place to learn, first-hand, about physicians' attitudes with respect to administrators and programs designed to control utilization and quality of care.[36]

The recent graduate of a health administration program taking a residency or entry-level position in a large hospital or health agency will probably be in a position to observe what an effective administrator does. Since this is a critical formative stage in one's career, it should provide the nascent administrator with an opportunity to find a role model on whom to pattern professional development. The fortunate beginner will have an opportunity to learn how experienced administrators set priorities without getting bogged down in administrivia; how they sift through reams of paper to keep important projects on schedule and on course; how they manage organizational conflict while maintaining high morale and productivity; how they delegate, while maintaining ultimate responsibility for the quality of the work product; and how they hold their key subordinates accountable. This is the period when the new administrator will need guidance and nurturing so that his or her energies are properly directed, talents and skills fully developed, and mistakes (which are inevitable) intelligently analyzed and corrected so as to avoid repetition in the future.

If the neophyte administrator is fortunate, he or she will develop friendships among peers, as well as among more experienced administrators, who will assume the big brother or sister role. These relationships should be sought after and cherished, not only because it is essential to have professional colleagues but also because it is from his or her colleagues that the new administrator learns how work really gets done in the organization's structure and how information is gathered and communicated at the point where the grapevine has its roots. Later on in the administrator's career, it will be his or her turn to assume the role of mentor, guide, and teacher for younger administrators, a role which can add measurably to the satisfaction in one's career no matter the field.

Certain courses are usually considered generic and necessary for all health administrators. In addition, a variety of special courses may prove especially useful for the quality assurance specialist, depending on the individual's focus (public health, business administration, public administration, or health planning, for example).

The following types of courses are recommended:

1. The study of the health care delivery system in historical perspective is essential: what it is now; political, social, and economic factors contributing to its development; its special characteristics; its financing; the health care system in the United States as compared with systems in other western countries; our problems, and alternative solutions that have been proposed and the reasons why they have or have not been adopted. As one health planner stated recently, "If you think the United States doesn't have a health care system, just try to change it."

2. The study of how public policy is formulated should be a basic requirement; how laws affecting health care services are introduced, enacted, and implemented; which committees of Congress and the state legislatures are concerned with health, and how the committees relate to each other and to the executive branches of government (the federal and state bureaucracies).

3. The student should take seriously courses relating health care to the American political system, especially with respect to the changing role of government in the financing and regulation of health services. (Passage in 1935 of the Social Security Act opened the way for governmental intervention, through social insurance, in the financing of health services for selected populations and, concomitantly, for setting standards and regulation of services provided and paid for out of public funds.)

4. Courses are recommended in budgeting or financial administration, as well as in organization theory, since the responsibility and authority for organizing and evaluating programs and developing and managing budgets has traditionally been the administrator's.

5. The need for courses in medical care evaluation or quality assessment is essential. Notwithstanding the wealth of available material on quality assurance, including approximately 1,000 studies and papers published in the last 50 years, few writings organize or categorize the material into a theoretical framework to guide the student.

Extremely useful to this administrator have been two courses which probably would not have been taken had she been given a choice. The first, methods in social research, dealt with, among other things, the basic elements of the scientific method, including how to state researchable or answerable questions (hypotheses), how to test them (research design), when and how to apply various research methods (observation, questionnaires, interviews), data collection (including primary and secondary sources), problems in research (bias, probability and sampling, validity and reliability), data analysis (statistical inference), and report writing. The most important contribution of the course was an understanding of the tools, limitations, and language of research. In addition, the course provided new skills applicable to quality assurance programs which were subsequently undertaken. These new skills have been enormously helpful in critically understanding and interpreting the increasingly sophisticated studies reported in the literature.

The other related areas of study were quantitative methods and electronic data processing. A significant portion of the quality assurance program administrator's work involves empirical data, and its measurement, processing, and analysis. It is nearly impossible for the administrator to function with full effectiveness without a working knowledge of the applicable methods of research, quantitative analysis, and computer technology.

For example, during a site visit to a hospital seeking delegated status for the performance of PSRO review functions, the hospital's quality assurance program administrator described the sampling method for selecting charts for inclusion in an MCE study of hysterectomy as random. After a little probing, the following was found: they would choose 50 charts out of a universe of several hundred, and would use every sixth chart from a list of chart numbers, generated by computer. We asked, "What happens if the designated chart is missing?" The answer was "The next chart is pulled." The program administrator apparently missed the significance of the question. Further investigation revealed that missing charts probably belonged to readmitted patients. Clearly, the omission of readmitted cases, quite possibly for a complication related to the original procedure, introduced bias and thus cast doubt on the reliability and validity of the study. Thus, the hospital was unable to identify variations from acceptable standards of quality practice, making the MCE study nothing more than a paper exercise.

Complicated data displays and computer printouts can be intimidating. The techniques of statistical analysis should be familiar to the health administrator seeking a career in quality assurance, since these can be used to mislead the uninitiated.

Moreover, frequent clashes over professional jurisdiction or turf occur in the health system, as elsewhere. Many examples exist in the area of patient services; for example, the ophthalmologist versus the optometrist, psychologist versus psychiatrist, podiatrist versus orthopedic surgeon, oral surgeon versus plastic surgeon, and others. Similar territorial problems have been observed between for instance, the private (JCAH) and the public (HHS) sectors, as well as within the public sector (PSRO versus state Medicaid agencies).

Data manipulation was illustrated during one such territorial conflict when a state Medicaid agency, operating under intense political pressure, submitted documentation regarding the superiority of its review system (established under state law) compared to the PSRO review system (authorized and funded under federal law). A comparison made by the state agency claimed to demonstrate that the state review system was more effective than the PSRO program in reducing hospital lengths of stay throughout the state, its purpose being to weaken the PSRO program, while strengthening that of the state agency. The document was released to the United States Senate Finance Committee and to the State Senate and Assembly, in order to convince the legislators to enact legislation, at both the federal and state levels, prejudicial to the PSRO program.

However, careful analysis of the imposing data displays revealed (1) that they were incomplete and inaccurate, representing, in some instances, periods when PSROs were not yet in existence, thereby precluding any legitimate comparison of the two systems; (2) that the data displays were highly selective, not including all areas and all hospitals, but only those data supporting the favored outcome, others being conveniently omitted; and (3) that the sources of data were not consistent for the two systems or the periods studied. The political paydirt for the state agency was high, however, and the legislators, convinced by a spurious study, were led to a wrong conclusion.

More important than any set of academic courses or appropriate residency or entry-level exposure is the need to develop a sense of who you are, and what you are for, both in terms of your career and in your personal life. Health administrators, whether in hospital administration, quality assurance, or any other position, will soon learn that choices need to be made and personal values developed, defined, and understood.

An example of such a need in this writer's experience arose in the form of an assignment given while at an academic medical center. The university hospital, like many of its counterparts in other parts of the country, was experiencing a shortage of available beds, especially for elective surgery for which there was a six- to eight-week waiting period. The governing board decided to expand the facility to accommodate the growing demand for certain specialized services, including a newly created open-heart surgery unit. A justification for the expansion program was required for submission to the regional planning council, and I was asked to develop a research strategy to support a certificate of need. New York State had one of the few programs in the country at the time requiring such certification. The project seemed to offer an opportunity for creative thinking.

It did not take long, however, for me to realize that the expansion, as projected, did not mesh with the facts and that it might create serious problems. Many questions needed to be asked and answered; for example, what impact would it have on an already overbedded area (known irreverently in hospital administration circles as bed pan alley)? What would happen to the new municipal hospital center, or to the affiliated hospital, rebuilt to replace an ancient landmark, which was about to open across the street from the medical center? What of the well-known problem, the generally declining census and lower occupancy rate in municipal hospitals? The municipal hospital involved appeared to be no exception.

Instead of justifying an expansion, a white paper was developed highlighting the unanswered questions raised by the proposed expansion program. Fortunately, the chief executive officers and others in the medical center administration were able to use the paper for extensive discussion with key decision makers who ultimately sought alternative solutions to the problem. However, this is not always the outcome when career and personal values clash.

What Personal Attributes Are Needed?

The health administrator as a quality assurance specialist needs an abundance of energy and perseverance, a high frustration tolerance, and a capacity to juggle many responsibilities and projects at one time. Personal and professional honesty and integrity, and the ability to get along with people are critically important attributes, while a sense of humor is helpful for comic relief when the going gets rough.

Quality assurance program administrators, as all who are in positions of authority or responsibility, must be able to take criticism and to distinguish between the constructive (from which they can learn) and the frivolous or malicious (which they must ignore). A program administrator must also share the credit when things go well and praise those who have contributed to the program's achievement(s) or success.

Most administrators have a sense of urgency about getting things done. If they are skilled in the art of management, they will communicate this sense to their subordinates without haranguing them. The administrator who can recruit and keep self-starting staff is fortunate indeed, since the desire to move forward to achieve program objectives will be shared at various levels in the organization, not only at the top.

The quality assurance specialist should probably be a born planner, for he or she must be able to anticipate the consequences of administrative actions or policies. This is especially true in quality assurance, since the review program for which the administrator is responsible may involve sanctions against physicians or hospitals, or denial of payment by federal or state agencies to physicians, hospitals, and other institutional providers, for care not deemed necessary or appropriate. The quality assurance program administrator will enjoy no more popularity than any other person in authority who administers a regulatory program. Doctors will be angry about outside interference with their usual and customary practice of medicine, while administrators will be furious about lost reimbursement and empty beds.

Every administrator hopes to exercise good judgment in carrying out his or her decision-making and problem-solving responsibilities. However, the leadership role often requires the administrator to possess the ability to analyze complex situations with incomplete information and to solve problems and make decisions under extreme time pressures and other constraints, sometimes in a highly politicized milieu.

The Rewards and Challenges

Quality assurance offers the individual seeking a career in health administration a special set of rewards. The choice of a career in health care is often motivated by the desire to work in a field of human services and to help improve the quality of life for people in need of such services, in this case health and hospital services.

A career in administration offers anyone who is so inclined an opportunity to use his or her special managerial and administrative skills to accomplish the purposes or mission of a program or organization in which he or she probably has a special belief, or to which he or she has made a professional commitment.

A career as a quality assurance specialist can combine human services with administration in the special field which seeks to correct or ameliorate many of the long-standing ills of the medical care delivery system. Such programs, whether conducted by public or private agencies or by providers of health services, are designed to assure that only services which meet professional quality standards and are medically necessary will be provided and paid for at the lowest cost consistent with the patient's needs. Since health care resources, both manpower and materiel, are finite, it should follow that quality assurance will improve the distribution of these limited resources and improve access to needed medical care for the total population.

One of the most satisfying aspects of this author's experience has been the sense of working at a frontier in health administration. Since PSROs are still relatively new and experimental in their methods and approaches, participation in the early implementation of one such program has presented a unique challenge, in part because we view the PSROs as change agents and as a major innovation in health care delivery in the United States. By establishing standards of practice, these agencies can, we believe, improve the quality of services provided by physicians and hospitals, reduce over-utilization and waste, and allow accountability.

In his 1975 essay, "Professional Self-Regulation in the Public Interest: The Intellectual Politics of PSRO," Scott Greer alluded to the possibility that "...the process of review may place PSROs in the position of highlighting unneeded treatment, as in tonsillectomy in children, and allow the physician to say 'No' with finality to the parents."[37]

One of the early findings of one PSRO appears to support this prediction. During the first year of its operations in a specialty hospital, the PSRO noted a 32 percent decrease in the number of tonsillectomies and adenoidectomies performed. By studying a comparable specialty hospital which was not yet under the PSRO review system, it was possible to determine that a statistically significant drop occurred in the PSRO hospital, which was not found in the non-PSRO hospital. Although the annual number of both these operations was declining in both hospitals, as it was in hospitals all over the country at a rate of approximately 5 percent annually for the three-year period prior to the beginning of the PSRO review program, the drop in the PSRO-reviewed hospital was much more dramatic (six times greater than in the non-PSRO hospital), confirming the hypothesis that PSRO can reduce the incidence of unnecessary surgery.

More important than any cost saving or reductions in unnecessary utilization which may result from review programs, such as those currently being performed under PSRO auspices, is the potential for identifying and correcting serious medical practice problems. The PSRO concurrent review system, by requiring trained nurses and physicians to scrutinize the chart of every federal admission to a hospital, provides a unique opportunity for quality review to be performed while the patient is still in the hospital. If effective, the review process allows the following questions to be addressed: Is the hospitalization necessary or could the care be provided on an outpatient basis? Is the diagnostic or surgical procedure necessary? Is the plan of treatment consistent with the diagnosis? Do the laboratory, x-rays, and other clinical tests and reports confirm the diagnosis and justify the treatment provided or planned? Is the necessary care being provided to the patient on a timely basis? Does the care provided during the patient's hospitalization meet professionally recognized standards?

During the first two years of operation, the New York County PSRO review system revealed that up to 20 percent of the patients admitted to particular hospitals could have been treated on an outpatient basis; that patients in some hospitals spent endless days as inpatients when no care was provided; that patients treated in a hospital for alcoholism left the hospital on pass days only to return intoxicated; that a battery of tests was ordered on all admissions to a major hospital, but that abnormal results were not appropriately followed up prior to every patient's discharge; that certain hospitals had unusually high mortality rates for no apparent reason; that a small group of physicians in a particular hospital accounted for the majority of surgical complications; and that these problems were known or suspected by their agencies, but that no corrective actions were ever required because they were difficult to document.

These problems are now being resolved. But if these revelations are any indication, the challenge to the quality assurance specialist health administrator will be to orchestrate the necessary responses from all the individuals and agencies which play a part in assuring the proper provision of health care services in the medical-hospital complex.

Conclusion

Recent federal legislation affecting health care financing programs has tended to incorporate and require quality and utilization controls based on methodologies of prototype review systems which have evolved during the last 60 years. The focus has been on increasingly objective methods of medical care appraisal. Moreover, the responsibility for effective implementation of medical quality assurance programs has come to be identified more and more with the health administrator's role as quality assurance specialist.

The PSRO review system represents the most ambitious attempt, to date, to establish effective, timely, and economical quality assurance mechanisms for the nation's health care delivery system. While the PSROs' initial efforts have been concentrated in short-term hospitals, the original legislation and its subsequent amendments require that these review systems be expanded into review of long-term care facilities and extended to cover ambulatory care settings. Although currently limited to federally financed programs, many PSROs are nonetheless undertaking review activities for the privately paid health sector.

PSROs have been subject to a number of studies, legal actions, congressional investigations, and professional debates of their viability and potential for true quality and utilization control. However, even if the PSRO program as it is now constituted should be discontinued, which some critics view as a distinct possibility, a form of quality control and evaluation is bound to be required not only under the current Medicare-Medicaid program but also under any planned national health insurance scheme.

Future quality assurance programs will be administered, whether by a centralized federal agency, or by a regional, state, or local governmental or quasigovernmental agency, or by private organizations (including, perhaps, insurance carriers or consumer organizations) operating under government contract, and therefore will require administrators who are prepared to assume responsibility for organizing, developing, managing, and implementing ongoing quality assurance programs in health care settings.

NOTES

[1]*Darling* v. *Charleston Community Memorial Hospital*, 33 Ill. 2d 326, 211 N.E.2d 253 (1965). See H.L. Kinser, legal counsel, Illinois Hospital Association, "Responsibility of Administration and Trustees for Medical Care," in *Proceedings of Institute on Legal Problems*, Catholic Hospital Association, St. Louis, 1967, for an analysis of the practical implications of the *Darling* case for trustees and administrators.

[2]For a full discussion of the *Darling* case vis-à-vis the evolution of public opinion on this subject, see Anne R. Somers, *Hospital Regulation: The Dilemma of Public Policy*, Chapter 2, Common Law, "Hospital Negligence and Responsibility for Quality Care." Princeton: Princeton University Press, 1969. pp. 28–37.

[3]While two earlier cases were settled by similar decisions (*Bing* v. *Thunig*, 2 N.Y.2d 656, 163 N.Y.S. 2d 3, 143 N.E.2d 3 [1957], and *Goff* v. *Doctors General Hospital of San Jose*, 166 Cal. App. 2d 314, 333 P.2d 29 [1958]), the *Darling* case is the one which is recognized for establishing the doctrine of corporate negligence.

[4]Anne R. Somers, *op. cit.* (note 2), p. 35.

[5]*Ibid.*

[6]Avedis Donabedian, M.D., *A Guide to Medical Care Administration; Volume II. Medical Care Appraisal—Quality and Utilization.* New York: The American Public Health Association, 1969.

[7]*Ibid.*, p. 1.

[8]Donabedian's theoretical framework for classifying approaches to medical care appraisal has been so widely accepted and used that recent articles in the literature no longer credit him with its conceptualization.

[9]Abraham Flexner, *Medical Education in the United States and Canada.* New York: Carnegie Foundation, 1910.

[10]Paul A. Lembcke, M.D., "Evolution of the Medical Audit." *Journal of the American Medical Association* 199 (1967): pp. 543–50.

[11]Ernest A. Codman, M.D., *A Study of Hospital Efficiency—The First Five Years.* Boston: Thomas Todd Co., 1916.

[12]Paul A. Lembcke, *op. cit.* (note 10).

[13]Ernest A. Codman, *op. cit.* (note 11).

[14]Paul A. Lembcke, *op. cit.* (note 10).

[15]*Ibid.*

[16]R. Heather Palmer, M.B., B. Ch., S.M. in Hyg., "Choice of Strategies," in Richard Greene, M.D., *Assuring Quality in Medical Care.* Cambridge, Massachusetts: Lippincott Co., 1976. p. 72.

[17]For an extensive description of the evolution and role of the JCAH in quality assurance, see Anne R. Somers, *op. cit.* (note 2).

[18]John D. Blum, Paul M. Gertman, and Jean Rabinow, *PSROs and the Law*, Chapter 1, "The Development of Peer Review." Germantown, Maryland: Aspen Systems Corp., 1977, pp. 1–17.

[19]Paul A. Lembcke, *op. cit.* (note 10).

[20]Odin W. Anderson, Ph.D., and Paul B. Sheatsley, *Hospital Use—A Survey of Patient and Physician Decisions.* Chicago: Center for Health Administration Studies, University of Chicago, 1967.

[21]*Ibid.*

[22]Donald C. Reidel and T.B. Fitzpatrick, *Patterns of Patient Care.* Ann Arbor: University of Michigan, 1964.

[23]Avedis Donabedian, *op. cit.*, (note 6) p. 21.

[24]U.S. Department of Health, Education and Welfare, Social Services Administration, *Health Insurance For the Aged/Conditions of Participation for Hospitals,* Washington, D.C., 1966.

[25]John D. Blum et al., *op. cit.* (note 18), p. 5.

[26]R. Heather Palmer, *op. cit.* (note 16), pp. 65–71.

[27]Paul A. Lembcke, "Measuring the Quality of Medical Care Through Vital Statistics Based on Hospital Service Areas: Comparative Study of Appendectomy Rates." *American Journal of Public Health* 42 (1952): pp. 276–286.

[28]Paul A. Lembcke, "Medical Auditing by Scientific Methods." *Journal of the American Medical Association* 162 (1956): pp. 646–55.

[29]*Ibid.*

[30]John W. Williamson, M.D., et al., "Continuing Education and Patient Care Research." *Journal of the American Medical Association* 201 (1967): pp. 938–42.

[31]Robert H. Brook, M.D., et al., "Assessing the Quality of Medical Care Using Outcome Measures: An Overview of the Method." *Supplement to Medical Care,* September 1977.

[32]Robert H. Brook, M.D., "Quality—Can It Be Measured?" *New England Journal of Medicine* 296 (1977): pp. 170–71.

[33]New trends in Continuing Medical Education identified by Robert K. Richards, Ph.D., American College of Cardiology, Bethesda, Maryland, were presented at the Alliance for Continuing Medical Education (ACME) Invitational Conference, Chicago, Illinois, February 1, 1978.

[34]Paraphrased from 42 U.S.C.A. § 1320c–4 (1977).

[35]David Kessner, M.D., "Quality Assessment and Assurance: Early Signs of Cognitive Dissonance." *New England Journal of Medicine* 298 (1978): pp. 381–86.

[36]Women administrators face special problems. Historically there has been a systematic exclusion of women in the United States from medical practice as well as from top-level positions, including those in hospital administration. It has been noted, for example, that only 9 percent of the nation's physicians are women (although, due to the women's movement, the percentage of female medical students is now rising).

As of 1974, their median income was about two-fifths that of equivalently educated male physicians. In addition, although 75 percent of all health workers are women, they are among the lowest paid groups in the nation. Therefore, women who seek careers in health administration as quality assurance specialists will need to be aware of the challenges they will face in the male-dominated medical care establishment.

[37]Scott Greer, Ph.D., "Professional Self-Regulation in the Public Interest: The Intellectual Politics of PSRO." In *Proceedings: Conference on Professional Self-Regulation.* U.S. Department of Health, Education and Welfare, PHS, June, 1975, p. 106.

180

15

As Health Insurance Administrator

Peter Rogatz, M.D., M.P.H., and Donald Meyers, B.S.

The patient is the first party—by convention and presumably by conviction the most important. The second party is the generic provider of health care services—the practitioner or the institution. The third party has become no less dispensable as payer of the bills rendered by the second party for services. Historically the third party was only grudgingly tolerated as an irritating but necessary interloper in the health care transaction. With good reason, providers feared that the third party would eventually feel its duties went beyond payment alone. The third party may be government (e.g., Title V, Medicare, Medicaid) or commercial health insurance or Blue Cross-Blue Shield—the most prominent nongovernmental, nonprofit third party. It is imperative to gain a sophisticated understanding of the role of health administrators in the workings of this health insurance spectrum.

The chapter by Peter Rogatz and Donald Meyers illustrates that administrators in health insurance institutions do considerably more than pay claims in a timely and accurate fashion. (L.E.B.)

Before we began writing this chapter, we discussed with considerable interest Dr. Lowell Bellin's invitation to contribute to this collection. What insights would we be able to bring to graduates of programs in health administration who might seek career opportunities in the field of health insurance?

First of all, since each of us has spent several years as an officer of Blue Cross and Blue Shield of Greater New York, we believe we have a solid understanding of the Blue Cross-Blue Shield system in general, and of its largest member Plans in particular. Second, our prior experience as hospital executives over a period of some 20 years has given us a thorough understanding of what third-party reimbursement means to hospitals in today's world. The two kinds of experiences in combination have given us an unusually good perspective on health insurance and its impact upon health care delivery in this country. Finally, in our current role as health care consultants, we have, in a sense, stepped back from the trees and find ourselves able to take a look at the forest. Standing outside of the day-to-day activities of both providers and third-party payers enables us to assume the perspective of the whole field, including the employment opportunities within it.

This chapter focuses primarily on the Blue Cross-Blue Shield system. However, since many other types of organization play significant roles in the overall field of health insurance, we have given some attention to these, pointing out important areas of contrast.

Role of Third Parties in Health Care Delivery

A general review of the history of health insurance in the United States will be helpful as background for the discussion which follows. The antecedents of health

---

Peter Rogatz, M.D., M.P.H., and Donald Meyers, B.S., are the principal members of the consulting firm which bears their names, Peter Rogatz & Donald Meyers Associates, Inc., of Roslyn Heights, New York.

insurance made their appearance in this country late in the nineteenth century, through the formation of mutual aid societies. In return for periodic payments, each member was entitled to cash benefits in the event of illness or accident. Soon thereafter, some insurance companies began to write policies for protection against specific illnesses; benefits were usually limited, and were related primarily to loss of income rather than to incurred costs of medical care.

The serious beginning of the health insurance movement in the United States came in 1929, when a group of schoolteachers developed a plan through an agreement with Baylor Hospital in Dallas which assured members of the provision of hospital services when needed in return for monthly payments made by the group. This arrangement, drawing heavily on the concept of a consumers' cooperative, proved extremely successful.

The onset of the Depression gave great impetus to the concept, which soon spread to other communities throughout the country and became the seed for the future Blue Cross system. Under the tremendous financial pressure of the Depression, hospitals were pleased to be able to make arrangements with large groups. The groups, in turn, sought to exercise effective bargaining power and assure themselves of hospital services at favorable rates. Individuals were protected against the risk of costly hospitalization and the institutions were protected against the hazard of bad debts. By the end of the 1930s, a number of Blue Cross Plans had been developed throughout the country. Soon thereafter, Blue Shield Plans providing coverage for medical and surgical expenses began to evolve.

The growing popularity of Blue Cross and Blue Shield Plans gradually elicited interest on the part of the commercial insurance companies. Initial estimates that the health insurance market was not worth entering were discarded during the 1940s; soon thereafter, insurance companies actively entered the market, offering coverages for hospital, medical, and surgical expenses.

A third category of independent health plans, very different from both the Blues and the insurance companies, also evolved. These were the prepaid group practice plans, whose roots may be traced back to the rural cooperatives of the late 1920s. Not until the 1930s and 1940s did a significant number of prepaid group practice plans develop in locations throughout the country, paving the way for the health maintenance organization (HMO) movement.

In the United States in 1975, a total of 165 million persons under the age of 65 had some type of health insurance protection. This number excludes persons over 65 (all of whom are covered as Medicare beneficiaries) and persons entitled to care under Title 19 of the Social Security Act (known in most states as the Medicaid program).

Of these 165 million, virtually all had protection for hospital expenses; approximately 96 percent had some type of surgical expense coverage, and approximately 92 percent had some type of coverage for regular medical expenses.

Of those with some type of hospital coverage, approximately half were covered by Blue Cross Plans, slightly more than half by insurance company policies, and just under 6 percent by independent plans. (In some instances there is duplicating coverage, so that the actual percentages add to somewhat more than 100 percent.)

Of persons having some type of surgical or medical expense coverage, about 44 percent were covered by Blue Shield Plans, about 56 percent by insurance company policies and just under 8 percent by independent plans.

Persons over the age of 65 are covered by Title 18 of the Social Security Act, the so-called Medicare program. In addition, certain designated categories of disabled persons are also covered under this program. As of July 1, 1975, more than 24 million persons were beneficiaries of the Medicare program. All of these had protection for hospitalization under the compulsory Part A element of the program, and more than 97 percent had protection for physicians' services under the voluntary Part B program, which requires a partial contribution by the covered individual. It is worth noting that almost 13 million of these Medicare beneficiaries had, in addition, supplementary protection either from Blue Cross and Blue Shield Plans (more than 8 million), from insurance company policies (just under 6 million), or from under independent plans (about 750,000).

The Medicaid program (Title 19 of the Social Security Act) permits each state to develop programs for hospital, medical, and related services for persons with incomes insufficient to pay for health care. Such programs, funded jointly by federal and state monies, provided services in fiscal 1975 for an estimated almost 23 million people.

Characteristics of the Major Third Parties

A brief review of the salient characteristics of each of the major third parties will illustrate their relative roles and the career opportunities they offer.

Blue Cross and Blue Shield Plans

These Plans are organized as special nonprofit corporations under the laws of the state in which they are located. As of June, 1978, there were 69 Blue Cross Plans and 70 Blue Shield Plans in the United States, each covering a specified geographic jurisdiction, with the Blue Cross Plans essentially providing coverage for hospital service and the Blue Shield Plans coverage for physicians' services. (Many of these Plans also sponsor HMOs and provide coverage for other important services such as dental care and prescription drugs, but in the interest of brevity these additional services will not be discussed here.)

In recent years there has been a significant trend toward combining Blue Cross and Blue Shield Plans into single organizations in order to provide greater efficiency and permit programmatic innovation. Of the 139 Plans, 37 of the 69 Blue Cross and 37 of the 70 Blue Shield Plans are now joined, so that the effective total of Blue Cross and Blue Shield Plans is 102. The separate Plans maintain varying degrees of cooperation; thus, even where two separate Plans exist there may be an agency agreement under which one Plan carries out on behalf of another certain basic support activities such as computer service, marketing, and so on.

The picture is a complex one, since Blue Cross Plans having jurisdiction over adjacent areas (whether or not within the same state) will compete with each other in the health insurance market. An employer with major offices in two adjacent states (or, for that matter, in two widely separated states) could obtain coverage from the Blue Cross Plan in either region, in which case that Plan would be responsible for paying benefits to covered members wherever they may live, as long as they are hospitalized in an institution that has a contract with some Blue Cross Plan.

Competition between the insurance companies and the Blue Cross and Blue Shield Plans is particularly keen for large national organizations whose health benefits plans embrace very substantial numbers of people living and working in different locations throughout the country. The problem of providing benefits for the employees of large corporations is somewhat simpler for the insurance companies, since their benefits are provided essentially in the form of cash indemnities, paid in accordance with a specified schedule upon presentation of receipted bills. By contrast, each Blue Cross Plan provides benefits in the form of hospital service rather than cash payment. Each Plan must establish and maintain agreements with hospitals throughout its area. Under such an agreement, a hospital contracts to provide specified types of services without charge to patients with Blue Cross coverage, and the Blue Cross Plan then pays the hospital for such services.

In order to compete effectively with the insurance companies in the provision of benefits to large nationwide purchasers, Blue Cross Plans, working together through the national Blue Cross Association, have devised a carefully designed series of inter-plan agreements. Any single Blue Cross Plan can assume responsibility as the control Plan, in order to underwrite large national accounts, with the assurance that service benefits will be delivered in any institution any place in the country which maintains a member agreement with any other Blue Cross Plan.

Because Blue Cross and Blue Shield Plans gain certain benefits from their non-profit status, they are regulated by one or more state agencies, most commonly either the Department of Insurance or the Department of Health, or both. Virtually every aspect of the operation of any Blue Cross or Blue Shield Plan is subject to regulatory control, including benefit structure; underwriting rules; rate making (setting of premium levels); development of formulae, rules, and schedules for reimbursement to hospitals, physicians, dentists, pharmacies, and other providers; calculation of specific payment rates to hospitals (application of previously approved formulae); contracts with hospitals and other providers; contracts with subscribers; and many other elements of the overall operation of Plans.

The social objectives of Blue Cross and Blue Shield Plans have been the subject of considerable debate, particularly in recent years. Critics point to the fact that the boards of directors of these Plans include hospital trustees, hospital executives, physicians, and other providers. These critics assert that Blue Cross and Blue Shield Plans are operated more for the benefit of providers than for the benefit of their subscribers. This argument has gained credence because for many years the boards of directors were dominated numerically, and probably philosophically, by providers.

However, an examination of trends in recent years suggests that this view, based on a historical stereotype, is a misleading oversimplification. In the past decade or so, the composition of Blue Cross and Blue Shield boards of directors has changed dramatically. In 1966, more than three quarters of all Blue Shield Plans had boards of directors in which physicians represented a majority. By contrast, in 1977, just over half of all Blue Shield Plans (accounting for about 62 percent of Blue Shield enrollment) had boards of directors in which physicians were in the minority.

It may be argued that nonprovider representatives of the general public, despite their numerical superiority on a board of directors, will commonly be swayed by the provider minority. Perhaps this occurs in some situations, but if our own personal experiences as former officers of a major Blue Cross and Blue Shield Plan are a reliable indicator, there is little to fear on this score. One of us regularly attended meetings of the Board of Directors of Blue Cross and Blue Shield of Greater New York over a period of several years, and never once observed a major policy issue in which physicians or hospital representatives were able to win or vote or maneuver the outcome on an issue in which they were in disagreement with the public representatives. It may be argued, of course, that domination of a board of directors by a powerful minority is accomplished in more subtle ways; this can certainly occur, but it was not a major element in the formation of policy during our tenure as officers of Blue Cross and Blue Shield of Greater New York.

To some extent, of course, the changing composition of Blue Cross and Blue Shield boards of directors is the result of public pressure from regulatory agencies, consumer groups, or both. This, however, is the way all institutions change in a democracy, and it does not seem to us to condemn the way these Plans are organized, but rather to affirm that they are flexible enough to respond constructively to social pressures.

Certainly, the growing number of instances of confrontation (and frequently litigation) between Blue Cross Plans and hospitals, and between Blue Shield Plans and physicians, suggests that these organizations are taking policy positions designed to protect the interests of their subscribers *vis-à-vis* the interests of providers. The time when relationships between the Blue Plans and their participating providers were relatively free of controversy has long since passed. It is common for hospitals to complain that they receive inadequate rates of payment from Blue Cross Plans and that services which they have provided in good faith are disallowed without sufficient reason. Hospitals have often resorted to lawsuits in the search for remedies to their conflicts with Blue Cross Plans. Physicians also have been lodging bitter complaints against Blue Shield Plans with increasing frequency.

In considering the relative roles of the Blue Plans, the insurance companies, and the independent plans within the overall context of health services in the United States, it helps to envision the three different categories of health insurance organizations as ranged along a spectrum in terms of consumer participation in policy formation, relationships with providers, and so on. Along this spectrum, the insurance companies tend to be the least concerned with consumer participation, the independent plans tend to be the most concerned, and the Blue Cross and Blue Shield Plans tend to occupy some sort of middle ground.

Traditionally, the insurance companies have dealt with their responsibilities very differently than have the Blue Plans. While Blue Cross Plans have been based upon the concept of service benefits, requiring the development and maintenance of agreements with hospitals, the insurance companies have provided benefits mainly in the form of cash indemnity, payable to the insured person upon submission of a receipted bill for services covered under his or her policy. Whereas Blue Cross Plans have commonly provided at least a portion of their coverage on a community-rated basis, so that poor risk groups can share the benefit of lower premiums through pooling with good risk groups, the insurance companies write their coverage on an experience-rated basis. Under the latter system, a group that has heavy utilization of benefits in one year will be required to pay a higher premium the following year (or soon thereafter); conversely, a group whose utilization is relatively low will receive a reduction in premium rates within a year or two. Under such a system, a third-party payer bears only limited financial risk and has relatively limited incentives to control improper utilization, to scrutinize claims, or to disallow claims if evidence of abuse is uncovered.

In the early stages of the health insurance movement, experience rating (which the authors personally consider a socially undesirable mechanism for the reasons stated above) was indeed confined largely to the insurance companies, and frowned upon by the Blue Plans. Large corporations, because of the age distribution and other characteristics of their employees, tend to have more favorable utilization experience than small groups. Thus, by utilizing experience rating, insurance companies were able to achieve a significant marketing advantage over the Blue Plans. As a result, a gradual trend developed in which the insurance companies were more likely to be selected for health care coverage by large corporations, leaving the Blue Plans with the smaller groups, which are associated with more costly administrative expenses and, quite often, higher rates of utilization. This, in turn, tended to drive the community-rated premiums applicable to smaller groups higher and higher. As a result, the Blue Plans began sometimes reluctantly and sometimes eagerly, to adopt experience rating; it is now a significant element in the marketing practices of many of the Plans.

The question of utilization review as a method for cost containment is another aspect of health insurance where the insurance companies and the Blue Plans have somewhat different characteristics, although not so strikingly different that one of them is branded the good guy, and the other the bad guy. To the extent that the Blue Plans have depended upon community rating and have been subject to closer regulatory scrutiny than the insurance companies, they have had a stronger incentive to develop effective claims review and utilization control. Experience rating tempts companies to pass costs along to the group purchaser, rather than to develop new programs for control of unnecessary utilization.

When pressures for utilization review developed in the mid-1960s in response to Medicare program regulations, the Blue Plans were not far ahead of the insurance companies. Because they serve as Medicare intermediaries more commonly than do the insurance companies, the Plans have moved more rapidly in the field of utilization review than the insurance companies. Only within the past few years have insurance companies moved in this direction, as spiraling health care costs have driven premiums so high that no organization—neither insurance company nor Blue Plan—can expect to pass the increased costs along to group purchasers in the form of another premium increase.

The differing nature of benefits—service benefits in the case of Blue Cross Plans, cash indemnity in the case of the insurance companies—has also compelled the Blues to develop utilization review and control more rapidly and to a somewhat higher level than the insurance companies. Confrontations occur more commonly when service benefits are involved and a Blue Cross Plan must say directly to a member hospital, "we believe you have provided unnecessary services and we will therefore not pay for them." Such confrontations with providers occur rarely in the case of insurance companies, since they make their payments to the insured individual rather than to the provider. When an insurance company disallows payment on the ground that a service was provided unnecessarily, the insured person becomes, to some extent, a buffer between the company and the provider, limiting the frequency and severity of confrontations.

Boards of directors of insurance companies are, understandably, concerned with profits. The formation of health insurance policy is closely related to whether selling such insurance coverage is profitable. Often the profit is only the indirect result of selling a package combining life insurance, pension, basic medical-surgical and hospital coverage, and major medical coverage. Under such conditions, the medical-surgical or hospital insurance may well be a loss leader, valued by the insurance company essentially as a marketing device. Thus, not only the question of utilization control but also fundamental issues such as consumer participation in policymaking, which have received considerable attention from the Blue Plans in recent years, have been of relatively less concern to insurance companies.

Independent Plans

At the other end of the spectrum are various independent health care plans. Space does not permit a full description of all of them, or even a summary classification. What will be presented here is a brief discussion of two major types of independent plans which both fall within the overall rubric of health maintenance organizations. The HMO concept was first officially enunciated by the Nixon administration in 1971, based upon the ideas of Dr. Paul Ellwood who originated the term "health maintenance organization." The concept, as articulated by Dr. Ellwood in 1971, refers to "...any organized system of health care that provides a full range of health maintenance and treatment services to an enrolled population in return for the prepayment of a fixed annual sum."

Without in any way detracting from the achievement of Dr. Ellwood, who is a most innovative and creative thinker, we can trace the two key forms of HMOs—prepaid group practice and individual practice associations—to pre-Nixon administration origins.

Prepaid Group Practice: Prepaid group practice plans can trace their historical origins at least as far back as 1929, with the establishment of the Ross-Loos Clinic in Los Angeles and the Farmers Union Hospital Association in Elk City, Oklahoma. Within the next decade or so, many of the organizations now well known as prepaid group practice plans were formed, including Group Health Association of Washington, D.C. (1937), Group Health Cooperative of Puget Sound (1945), and the Health Insurance Plan of Greater New York (1947). The best known and most successful prototype, the Kaiser Foundation-Permanente Medical Care Program, was established around 1950.

In the prepaid group practice model, the physicians are organized as a medical group, practicing in a common facility, sharing professional income and professional expenses. The medical group is at risk concerning the utilization of health services by subscribers and the total cost of the program.

Individual Practice Association: The IPA concept traces its origins back to the San Joaquin Foundation for Medical Care, which was organized in 1954. This plan, clearly the prototype for the IPA version of HMO, was designed as an alternative to the rapid development of prepaid group practice through the Kaiser-Permanente plan in California. In contrast to the group practice arrangement, this model provides that the physicians continue to function as solo practitioners (or, if they prefer, in small, independent groups). An HMO is formed which, through a set of agreements with a corporation, association, or some other legal entity, contracts with physicians (and other providers such as dentists and optometrists). The individual providers may or may not be at risk in this model, depending upon the type of reimbursement arrangements which the IPA has made with them.

Both HMO models provide comprehensive health services to enrolled persons in exchange for an annual prepaid fee; by placing the providers at risk for the utilization and cost of medical services, this arrangement gives the providers an incentive to promote health, to prevent illness, and to diagnose, treat, and rehabilitate sick persons as promptly and effectively as possible.

The very substantial differences between HMOs as health insurers and the more conventional Blue Cross and Blue Shield Plans or commercial insurance companies are readily apparent. HMOs differ among themselves with respect to the comprehensiveness of services provided, the use of coinsurance provisions, the arrangements for provision of hospital services, and various other significant factors. However, in all instances, the HMO concept involves a much closer relationship between consumers and providers, with much greater attention to the way health services are provided, the utilization characteristics of enrolled persons, the possibility of overutilization or abuse, and other elements central to the health care delivery process itself. This is even more characteristic of the prepaid group practice plans than it is of the independent practice associations.

The growth of health maintenance organizations was disappointingly slow during the early years of the 1970s. In 1971, when Dr. Ellwood's concept was first adopted, there were 33 such organizations in the United States. By 1973, despite the enthusiastic urgings of the Nixon administration, this number had grown only to 42, serving a total of some 4 million persons. In December, 1973, federal legislation (P.L. 93–222) was enacted to stimulate HMO development. The movement gained momentum thereafter, and by the end of 1977, some 165 health maintenance organizations were providing care to a total of some 6.3 million persons.

A Closer Look at One Blue Cross Plan

In 1934 Governor Herbert Lehman of New York signed legislation enabling the United Hospital Fund, supported by The Commonwealth Fund and the Josiah Macy, Jr., Foundation, to work for the creation of Associated Hospital Service of New York— the Blue Cross Plan that would serve New York City, Long Island, and the ten counties immediately north of New York City. This would eventually become the largest Blue Cross Plan in the United States, serving almost nine million subscribers.

As in the case of other Blue Cross Plans, Associated Hospital Service of New York (AHS) was organized with the active support and participation of the individual hospitals throughout the community. Fundamental principles embodied in the organization of AHS included the following:

AHS would seek to market hospital benefits to as broad a segment of the community as possible.

AHS would attempt to develop a premium level that would permit orderly growth and development.

AHS would pay to each participating hospital a per diem rate judged adequate and reasonable; each hospital would accept as payment in full the monies obtained through subscribers' premiums and would guarantee to deliver to AHS subscribers all ordinary hospital services without additional charge. This represented the critical service benefit concept, the heart of the social contract between subscriber, third-party payer, and participating provider institution, which was to be the foundation of all Blue Cross Plans.

AHS, along with its sister Blue Cross Plans throughout the country, grew slowly throughout the Depression and the years immediately preceding U.S. involvement in World War II. By the year 1940, enrollment in all Blue Cross Plans throughout the country totaled only about 6 million persons.

The decade immediately following the war saw an explosive growth in the provision of health care benefits for employed groups. Blue Cross enrollment skyrocketed from 6 million in 1940 to 19 million in 1945 and 51 million in 1955. Blue Shield enrollment in these same three years jumped from 370,000 to 3 million and then to 39 million. In the next two decades growth continued, although at a somewhat slower rate, bringing total enrollment to the levels described earlier in this chapter.

The history of AHS is particularly instructive with reference to its method of reimbursing member hospitals. The original, relatively simple arrangements with hospitals gave way to more complex and more restrictive methods of reimbursement. During the 1950s, AHS reimbursed each member hospital on the basis of a fixed per diem payment, adjusted periodically to reflect increases in the Bureau of Labor Statistics cost indexes. Despite the periodic adjustments, many hospitals were not able to recover the full cost of providing services to AHS subscribers.

In 1960 AHS introduced a very significant change in its payment method, designed to assure each hospital that it would be reimbursed the reasonable cost for provision of necessary services to subscribers, subject, however, to certain significant limitations. The methodology developed by AHS for calculating its reimbursement rates received wide circulation and played a significant part in the development of the methodology adopted by the federal Medicare program when that program was instituted in 1965. Under the reimbursement provisions instituted in 1960, AHS specified the services covered in its subscriber contracts, defined the cost components deemed necessary and appropriate for provision of these services, and established a retrospective method for adjusting per diem reimbursement, based upon a cost audit.

At the same time, AHS began to develop certain cost limitations to prevent its member hospitals from incurring excessive or inappropriate costs. Hospitals were placed in peer groups, and limitations were based upon the average costs within each peer group. Another type of limitation was based on each hospital's own rate of cost increase, with a limit on its annual rate of increase derived from its average rate of increase for the three prior years.

The introduction of the 1960 reimbursement methodology marked a significant milestone in the evolution of the Blue Cross philosophy, which involved a gradual but significant metamorphosis in relationships between the Plan and its provider institutions. Initially, AHS had been viewed as an instrument of the hospitals. Gradually, however, the Plan began to assume increasing responsibility for protecting the interests of its subscribers and began to see itself acting as a fiduciary agent on their behalf.

The problems of cost control, while recognized during the early 1960s, did not assume frightening proportions until after the middle of the decade. One of the most critical factors in fueling rapid cost increases was the passage of Titles 18 and 19 of the Social Security Act in 1965, creating the Medicare program (effective July 1, 1966), and the Medicaid program (effective January 1, 1966). The introduction of these two programs assured that very large populations previously uninsured or underinsured—the aged and the poor—suddenly became entitled to a wide range of hospital, medical, and other health services. Since the passage of Titles 18 and 19, these groups have obtained greater access to health services and have used these services with much greater frequency than they did previously, and with greater frequency than do persons under 65 years of age or persons gainfully employed.

This is not to suggest that these higher utilization rates are inappropriate—we believe they are quite justifiable—but rather to call attention to the very considerable expansion of demand that has occurred since 1966. This increased demand, coupled with the sudden infusion of additional funds available to pay for health services under Titles 18 and 19, fueled an inflationary spiral that, except for a temporary slowdown during the economic stabilization program in the early 1970s, has swept through the entire country and has proved frighteningly resistant to control. Methods of achieving constructive control have engaged the minds of thoughtful professionals throughout the health care system in the United States, and have become a major concern of Blue Cross and Blue Shield Plans and all other third-party insurers.

Some indication of the significance of the Medicare program in the overall pattern of health services in this country can be inferred from a review of the situation in New York. Blue Cross and Blue Shield of Greater New York is the Medicare Part A intermediary for the great majority of hospitals in the 17 counties that comprise its service area, and the Medicare Part B carrier for physicians in all but one of the 17 counties.

The impact of this relationship on the administrative and claims processing functions of the organization is impressive. In 1977 the Blue Cross-Blue Shield Plan paid approximately 1.8 million hospital claims (more than half of these for outpatient services) on behalf of subscribers under the age of 65; 3.6 million claims for basic medical-surgical and major medical coverage; and another 2.5 million claims for dental services and prescription drugs. In addition, the Plan processed 1.5 million claims in its role as Medicare Part A intermediary; 8 million claims as Part B carrier; and 1 million claims for supplementary Medicare coverage (underwritten and marketed directly by the Plan itself). Thus, about half of the claims processed by Blue Cross and Blue Shield of Greater New York in 1977 were on behalf of Medicare beneficiaries. Although the Medicare responsibility does not involve underwriting and risk taking, it clearly is a very substantial activity that has significantly enlarged the scope and responsibility of the New York Blue Cross-Blue Shield Plan.

This point can perhaps be made most effectively by viewing the New York Blue Cross Plan from an autobiographic perspective. The authors of this chapter joined that organization in the early 1970s, after each of us had spent some 20 years in various administrative positions in the health care provider field. These included significant leadership roles in prepaid group practice, community hospitals, teaching hospitals, and the medical school environment. Prior to joining the New York Blue Cross Plan, Peter Rogatz served as Associate Director of the Health Sciences Center of the State University of New York at Stony Brook, as well as Professor of Community Medicine; Donald Meyers served as Director of the University Hospital and Assistant Professor of Health Services Administration.

What was it that attracted the two of us to the New York Blue Cross Plan at a time when we were participating in the planning and growth of a major new health complex—schools of medicine, nursing, dentistry, allied health professions, social welfare and basic sciences, and the associated university hospital? Since the purpose of this chapter is to assist the reader in career planning, we believe it is important to summarize the key factors that moved us from the provider world to the payer world.

The payer world problems we encountered would be no less challenging than those we had experienced as executives in the provider field, and certainly no less complex. A Blue Cross Plan must be extremely sensitive to its responsibility as fiduciary agent for the premiums paid by its subscribers. It must not disenfranchise its subscribers nor in any way circumscribe benefits to which they are entitled. It must find ways to control costs, and it has immense power to do so. However, this power must be used carefully so as not to jeopardize inappropriately either subscribers or member institutions. Long-standing agreements with its provider institutions must be reviewed at regular intervals to ensure that they are serving the best interests of Plan subscribers, without creating conditions that are damaging and unacceptable to member institutions.

The challenge to seek opportunities for constructive change while honoring contractual commitments to providers and fiduciary responsibilities to subscribers—was an exciting one. Although the details have changed somewhat in the past several years, the fundamental challenges have not. They are typical of the many opportunities in the field of health insurance for persons with training in health administration. One of us (PR) was invited to join the Plan as senior vice-president, and the other (DM) to recruit and manage the small group of health professionals who would become the cadre for the development of new programs. A closer look at some of our experiences and activities in the New York Blue Cross Plan should help the individual considering a career in Blue Cross-Blue Shield administration to visualize the types of opportunities that may be available in such an environment. Some of the programs described below were originated many years before our association with the Blue Cross Plan, but we developed them; others were initiated during our tenure.

The New York Blue Cross Plan has, for many years, recognized its potential for constructively influencing health care delivery. As far back as the 1950s the Plan supported the landmark experiment in hospital-based home care at Montefiore Hospital and Medical Center in the Bronx. Success with this demonstration led Blue Cross to develop a home care benefit available to its subscribers on a communitywide basis. This has resulted in widespread diffusion of home care programs throughout the New York area. As of early 1978 there were some 37 hospital-based home care programs and 14 free-standing home care agencies that had entered into agreements with Blue Cross and Blue Shield of Greater New York to provide home health services for its subscribers, or on behalf of Medicare beneficiaries (for whom the Blue Cross-Blue Shield Plan acts as intermediary).

Another benefit innovation developed many years ago by the New York Blue Cross Plan as an alternative to hospital care was the provision of posthospitalization benefits in nonacute extended care facilities. Complex issues arise in this connection, particularly in the face of an acknowledged surplus of hospital beds. An important aspect of our Blue Cross responsibilities was some assessment of the extent of the bed surplus in the New York area and the development of approaches to this problem.

Blue Cross Plans throughout the country have been attentive to the potential inherent in the health maintenance organization concept for favorably influencing health care delivery. More than half of the Plans are sponsoring or are otherwise actively involved with health maintenance organizations. Efforts along these lines began at New York Blue Cross in 1970; soon after joining the Blue Cross Plan, Donald Meyers assumed responsibility for the project. Planning, analysis, and a careful set of negotiations led eventually to an agreement with one of the Blue Cross member hospitals—an outstanding teaching institution—to develop a model prepaid group practice program, marketed (and, initially, subsidized) by Blue Cross and Blue Shield of Greater New York.

In 1964 the New York Blue Cross Plan embarked upon another innovative effort—unique in the United States—involving an agreement with the Community Blood Center of Greater New York. Under this agreement the Blue Cross Plan paid the costs of blood processing for any blood transfusion given to one of its subscribers, if that subscriber (or a significant percentage of the subscribers enrolled in his or her organization) had previously donated blood and thereby secured a credit from the Community Blood Center. This program, which has proved to be an outstanding success over the years, has not only stimulated voluntary blood donation but also assured that the Blue Cross Plan will be paying for blood on behalf of its subscribers in a particularly economical way.

The Blue Cross activities in cooperation with the Community Blood Center gave rise to yet another innovative program—an arrangement with the New York Metropolitan Chapter of the National Hemophilia Foundation that resulted in the creation of an alternative benefit that pays for ambulatory treatment of hemophiliac patients. The availability of this benefit has not only facilitated patient care but also resulted in substantial savings to the Plan.

In 1972 the Blue Cross Plan initiated coverage for chronic kidney dialysis provided either on an ambulatory basis or at home for subscribers suffering from end stage renal disease. Although this innovation was soon rendered obsolete by the Social Security Amendments of 1973 (HR-1) which provided like coverage for all victims of end stage renal disease under the Medicare program, Donald Meyers's expertise in this area led to his participation in a task force organized by the Bureau of Health Insurance to aid in implementation of the new Medicare dialysis program.

In addition to these and other programs designed to affect the health care delivery system by broadening benefits, we recognized the opportunity at Blue Cross to effect change in connection with review and control of utilization. One such approach was the development of statistical analyses of the hospital experience of Blue Cross subscribers, for each hospital and each peer group, analyzing length of stay (average, median, and frequency distribution) by diagnosis and age group.

We were both actively involved in various other efforts concerned with improving the quality and scope of hospital data. Thus, Peter Rogatz became a member of a multi-agency consortium established to develop uniform data on hospital and health services throughout the State of New York. Donald Meyers played a major role in advising a local organization concerning its proposal for designation as a Professional Standards Review Organization (PSRO); these activities led subsequently to his becoming a member of that PSRO's Board of Directors.

Many occasions arose in our Blue Cross and Blue Shield roles for the application of our prior experiences as providers. As a result of the findings reported by Dr. Eugene McCarthy of Cornell University, Peter Rogatz proposed offering to subscribers for whom elective surgery had been recommended the provision without charge of a second opinion from a qualified specialist. This program, after a slow beginning, has gradually gained subscriber acceptance; it seems likely that the concept will, before long, be applied by third-party payers throughout the country (including Medicare).

At Blue Cross and Blue Shield of Greater New York, the Division of Provider Reimbursement has direct responsibility for developing reimbursement methodology and establishing rates of payment. Appeals are handled with joint input from the Legal Department and the Division of Health Affairs. The authors' input into the various activities of the Division of Provider Reimbursement included participation in negotiations concerning the reimbursement methodology, participation in analysis of appeal problems, and, perhaps most important, a role in the development of new reimbursement experiments.

Thus far we have focused attention on the relationship of third-party payers to providers. However, during our years at Blue Cross and Blue Shield of Greater New York we became increasingly sensitive—as did others across the nation—to the vital role that can and should be played by the individual in caring for his or her own health. Our concern with this long-neglected issue led us to propose an active health education program, one that would serve not only Plan subscribers but also the community at large. The response was favorable and such a program was established by Blue Cross and Blue Shield of Greater New York.

Throughout our activities in the third-party environment, we each retained a keen sense of our origins in the provider world. It was important to walk a fairly narrow line between extremes, either of which would have been a very serious error. On the one hand, we rejected the idea of abandoning our provider roots for the role of antiprovider turncoats; on the other hand, we rejected the role of being the provider mouthpiece within the Blue Cross and Blue Shield setting, merely serving as an internal mechanism for articulating the views of hospitals, physicians, and other providers.

In our view, what was and still is needed within the Blue Cross-Blue Shield system is a staff of people who have knowledge and experience of the workings of the provider world, people who are committed to the fundamental objectives of the Blue Cross-Blue Shield system but who are able to bring their provider knowledge to bear on the solution of problems requiring an understanding of both provider and third-party environments.

Through our activities in the Blue Cross-Blue Shield system we have developed the conviction that working in the third-party environment is just as important to health care delivery in this country as working in a health care institution. Of course, when a hospital executive becomes an officer of any third-party payer organization, he or she must reliquish identities and loyalties associated with a specific institution, but that officer need not and should not forget the principles and practices involved in running a hospital or caring directly for patients. It is just this knowledge and understanding that helps to generate excitement, innovation, and creativity within a third-party organization.

Tasks and Assignments in the Blue Cross Environment

The program graduate who has had experience in some of the more conventional areas of health administration will find the health insurance field to be a surprising mixture of the familiar and the unfamiliar. Activities involving interface between a Blue Cross Plan and its member hospitals, for example, is an area in which someone with prior hospital administration experience would readily find his or her way. By contrast, the actuarial and rate-making functions, which are of key importance in the health insurance field, would probably be *terra incognita* for most seasoned hospital or public health administrators.

A brief outline of the major activities which must be carried out by any Blue Cross or Blue Shield Plan or commercial insurance company will illustrate the range and the variety of tasks involved. These include the actuarial function (premium rate determination); the reimbursement function (establishing payments to providers); claims processing (determination of whether the claimant is an eligible insured person, whether the service is covered by the policy, whether benefits have been exhausted, just what benefit should be paid against each specific claim, and so on); interfacing with providers and developing and implementing policy with reference to various provider issues; legal affairs; marketing; and a variety of other activities essential to keep the house functioning and in order (computer, personnel, communications, and public relations, for example).

Theoretically, the graduate of a program in health administration who moves into the field of health insurance administration might become directly involved with any of the various activities outlined above. However, many of these functions require specific professional or technical preparation quite different from that provided to the graduate in health administration. From a practical point of view, it is likely that graduates of such programs would have jobs in the area of provider affairs or claims administration, and a somewhat more detailed outline of these areas may be of interest.

Responsibilities in the area of claims administration include the following:

Determination of whether the individual is covered under a policy issued by the Blue Cross-Blue Shield Plan or insurance company and whether that coverage was in effect at the time the services were provided;

Determination of whether the services provided are within the scope of benefits to which the individual is entitled under his or her contract or policy;

Determination of whether benefits have been exhausted;

Decision on whether to approve or disapprove the claim and, if the decision is to approve, determination of what benefits should be paid, followed by authorization to make payment.

Responsibilities in the area of provider affairs would include the following:

Maintenance of effective communications with all providers (institutions and pri-

192

vate practitioners) through their professional organizations (local and state medical societies and hospital associations) in order to communicate basic policies, procedures, and regulations;

Maintenance of direct, one-to-one contact with institutions and individual providers in terms of responding to requests for information, handling problems in regard to procedural rules, discussing policy issues, and so on;

Development and continuing review of contractual agreements with providers (for example, member hospitals, participating physicians, and dentists);

Participation in development of provider reimbursement policies;

Participation in the provider appeal process;

Participation in the development of policy in connection with benefit structure, program innovation, alternative delivery systems, and other issues dealing with Plan-provider relationships.

Utilization review and control fall within the purview of claims administration in some organizations and of provider affairs in other organizations. This function calls for the development and maintenance of effective data collection and analysis systems that make it possible to review claims and identify, from among the great volume of material, those claims that may represent improper utilization or abuse, by either the provider or the subscriber. Because of the very large number of individual claims involved, this almost inevitably requires the application of screening criteria which can, at an acceptable cost, identify suspicious claims. These, in turn, can be subjected to a series of increasingly precise screens or review processes, leading eventually to the identification of specific claims that should be disallowed, either in whole or in part.

Although the disallowance of specific claims in which there is evidence of abuse by subscriber or provider is an important and necessary activity, a more important objective should be to deter chronic offenders from continuing their abusive practices. A key measure in such an effort might be the identification, through statistical pattern analysis, of providers who are found to be chronic offenders. In such instances, deterrent or punitive measures directed specifically at a few conspicuous abuses should be of greater benefit both to the Plan and to its subscribers at large than the mere disallowance of specific individual claims.

The Blue Cross-Blue Shield environment offers many opportunities for individuals with varying education, interests, and skills. Men and women with backgrounds in health economics, health care planning, health care administration, medical-legal affairs, and health education may all find useful and professionally satisfying careers in the Blue Cross-Blue Shield system. Persons with knowledge and experience in governmental program management will also find that their skills are transferable to and valuable in the health insurance field.

Concluding Comments

Each of us found his way into exciting and rewarding roles in the Blue Cross-Blue Shield system after having spent many years in hospitals and other provider settings.

Of course, this career pattern is not the only way for someone professionally trained in health administration to enter the field of health insurance. There are many examples of individuals who have begun their careers in the health insurance field and have spent their entire professional lifetimes in that setting, making outstanding contributions and becoming illustrious leaders. There is no single path to success and productivity in the health insurance field.

We do believe, however, that Blue Cross and Blue Shield Plans should include among their senior executive personnel at least some individuals who have become seasoned in the provider world—as hospital managers, physicians, dentists, nurses,

193

and others who have had the experience of responding to the needs of patients. The cross-fertilization of ideas that takes place under such conditions must inevitably work to the advantage of the insurance plan, the providers, and, most important of all, the public at large. If there is one lesson that the two fo us believe we have learned and would like to pass along to others, it is the importance of third-party payers (Blue Cross and Blue Shield Plans and insurance companies) and providers (hospitals, nursing homes, physicians, dentists, and others) placing their own needs in proper perspective—which is to meet the needs of patients, consumers, and the general public.

This lesson, which some in the health care field apparently have yet to learn, is the single most important unifying concept that has given meaning to our careers for some 20 years as providers and for several years thereafter as third-party payers. It is the single most important thing that providers and third parties should recognize in common, and it should be the touchstone of all of their efforts.

16   As Financial Manager

Raymond J. Cisneros, C.P.A., F.H.F.M.A.

European critics have labeled the United States a mercantile society, or, more sneeringly, a nation of shopkeepers. Such name calling has not bothered Americans much. True, Americans through-out the 50 states share the cultural expectation that individuals are obliged somehow, sometime, to pay for everything, even for activities designed to help relieve suffering, such as the delivery of personal health services. Devoted as they may be to the well-being of patients, health workers still insist on being paid on time. There is no need, then, to be defensive about the consequent growth in influence of the financial manager whose skills can maximize the purchasing and earning potential of every dollar that enters the institutional pool. Omnicompetence in fiscal affairs is the prerequisite for institutional survival. Economic Darwinism dooms hospitals with inept financial management to bankruptcy, even though these hospitals may be otherwise fit professionally.

Raymond J. Cisneros has exemplary experience in the financial management of complex health care institutions. He presents an overview of the extraordinary range of responsibilities of today's sophisticated financial manager in health administration. (L.E.B.)

Introduction

The indispensable role that finance plays in the management of the modern health care institution focuses deserved attention on the administrator who serves as the institution's financial manager. In the past the financial manager with ambition to advance might have been expected to harbor secret yearnings for the top managerial post in the institution. In contrast, today financial management itself has become so complex and intellectually rewarding in its own right that the typical financial manager remains sufficiently well-challenged and content within his or her own locus of professional activity.

History of the Field

Before the advent of Medicare, the typical hospital relied more on gifts for acquiring funds than on maximizing business opportunities and business operations. In smaller hospitals the bookkeeper was the most experienced full-time finance person on the payroll; an outside accountant might have furnished supplementary services. In hospitals that had accounting staffs, financial activities rarely transcended the collection of bills and historical financial reporting. The institution, particularly the non-profit type, was viewed by others and by itself as a social or community agency rather than a business entity.

Raymond J. Cisneros, C.P.A., F.H.F.M.A., is former Vice-President for Financial Operations at the Affiliated Hospital Center, Inc., of Boston, Massachusetts. He is at present an audit partner of Touche, Ross & Co., also of Boston.

Larger institutions generally broke the ground for more sophisticated financial management. As Blue Cross adopted more of a negotiating stance, it was logical that more people with substantive backgrounds in finance be recruited for hospital staffs. By 1946 there were enough finance professionals in the health field to form an organization known as the American Association of Hospital Accountants. That organization, subsequently renamed the Hospital Financial Management Association, has grown from fewer than 200 original members in 1946 to 19,000 in 1980, and has led the field in the development of expertise in financial management.

Hospital salaries for nonphysicians before 1965 were relatively low, and fringe benefits minimal. The hospital pharmacy lacked today's extensive formulary. Long-term debt for construction was undertaken in only a few instances. The enactment of Medicare and Medicaid profoundly altered the financial future of hospitals. The flow of dollars into the health care system called more attention to the financial affairs of the health care institution. Limits and controls became more financially oriented. More stringent governmental requirements for billing and other financial activities expanded the requirements for financial documentation and processing. As a consequence, a greater number of financial employees were needed to cope with the increase in the overall hospital work force and the purchases that the newly founded Medicare and Medicaid funds now supported. Specialists in many areas within financial management became a necessity.

Thus the financial operations of the American hospital have been transformed from the simple and small to the large and complex. The hospital's financial operations now demand the application of sophisticated techniques not too dissimilar from those of corporate entities in the profit-making sector.

Background of a Financial Manager

The financial manager of several years ago came from varied backgrounds— sometimes from those unrelated to hospitals. The rapid growth of hospitals and the influence of business people on their governing boards provided impetus for stronger financial operations. Some finance personnel were recruited directly from profit-making industry into the health care field in an effort to inculcate businesslike management into the financial activities of the hospital. Such an individual would typically have the title of Controller, and, in the beginning at least, would rarely be viewed as a bona fide member of the management team. Sometimes an individual might have been hired from the accounting firm that had audited the hospital.

When the enactment of Medicare magnified the reimbursement function, strong financial management within hospitals became indispensable. The influx of people with superior technical accounting abilities into the health care field notwithstanding, there continued to be a shortage of seasoned and expert financial managers.

Today the field of hospital finance has matured to the point of developing its own leadership through a combination of formal didactic training and in-house, hands-on apprenticeship experience. The future financial manager enters the health care field with at least a baccalaureate if not a master's degree; he or she will be paid a salary competitive with those in general industry, will receive substantial fringe benefits, and can anticipate an upwardly mobile career ensured by the hospital's constant need for financial managers of quality.

The financial manager has moved stepwise from the position of controller, just outside the management team, to a position inside the management team, first as an assistant administrator, then as an associate administrator or vice-president of finance. In most health care institutions, the chief financial officer occupies the post of the number two or three person. The senior financial manager has become as critical to the hospital organization as the senior financial manager is to any public corporation. In the proprietary hospital, the chief executive officer may be a financial manager, reflecting the emphasis on the profitability of such enterprises. Figure 16-1 shows a representative hospital financial organization chart.

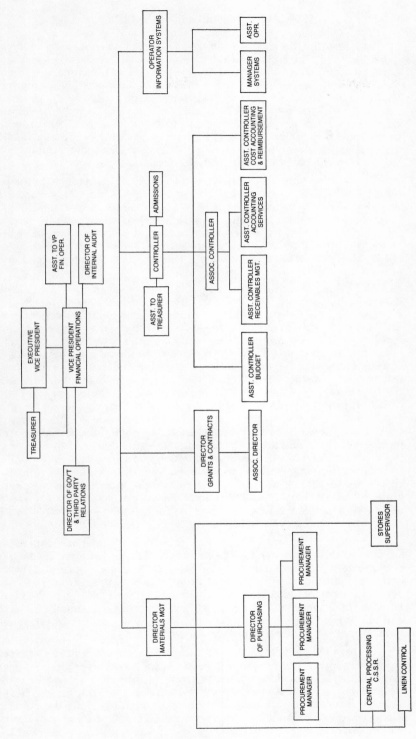

FIGURE 16-1

ORGANIZATION CHART
FINANCIAL OPERATIONS

197

Problems of the Field

Paradoxically, the problems of the field began when its fiscal problems appeared to be declining. The right-to-health-care movement, legislatively translated into Medicare, Medicaid, and Hill-Burton benefits, helped fuel inflationary health care costs. In the financing of expanded and new hospital facilities, the Hill-Burton program gave rise to larger facilities that were to add new hospital staff to the payroll. Equipment standards and the high level of health care services in publicly subsidized health delivery programs encouraged hospitals to spend more dollars in order to qualify for these funds. This phenomenon characterized particularly those hospitals whose patient populations were predominantly the aged and the indigent, those who had been least able in the past to pay for such services and improvements.

At the same time, the health care system began to unionize. In the past, hospital employees had been poorly paid. The conventional assumption seemed to be that such employees were to be altruistically devoted to their responsibilities. In effect, hospital employees had been contributing a portion of their salary potential toward the hospital's operation. With the onset of Medicare and Medicaid, hospital employees concluded that the traditional constraints against higher, more realistic wages had vanished. Moreover, a favorable economic climate in the country helped encourage this attitude.

The result? Health care costs rapidly rose. Medicare and Medicaid suffered cost overruns that had a formidable fiscal impact on the federal budget. Controls were introduced at the federal level in an attempt to constrain the acceleration of costs. At the state level with Medicaid, in those states with the most generous programs, fiscal constraints were imposed without necessary attendant cutbacks in client eligibility, benefits, and programs. Problems were compounded during the late 1970s when the country experienced a combination of economic inflation and recession. The health care industry was not isolated from the nation's climate, but it had hitherto rarely felt the impact other industries had. Inflation certainly reflected itself in the expenditure of health care dollars. The health care dollar as a percentage of the gross national production also grew, approaching 10 percent, in response to the growth and greater utilization of services, to an increasing staff-to-patient ratio, and to more complex and more expensive technology. There were increasing demands to stop or at least slow down accelerating health care costs. Budgetary constraints were translated into arbitrary limits to be imposed on the amount to be paid for certain services. Reimbursable costs were specified. The types and amounts of services covered were cut back. Some limits were established, although accompanying supportive study was inadequate; others were subsequently set aside by the courts; others were left intact. The attempt at rational planning entered the health care field belatedly.

Regrettably, the current planning process has sometimes turned out to be as arbitrary as the previously described cutbacks. Relatively uninformed neophytes from outside the health care field have occasionally formulated plans for health care and imposed them on the providers of care, with little input from those providers. A pervasive sense of helplessness has held sway in the face of increased hospital costs. Thus, approaches to cutting costs that have appeared academically sound have sometimes been tried with disastrous results. Others will doubtless disagree with my pessimistic analysis of much of health planning today.

Aware of the political reaction to its decisions, government has become hesitant to explicitly ration services to those in need of care. Government has indirectly imposed that task on the providers of care by reducing their resources without reducing the services they are expected to provide. Presumably, government and health care officials are increasingly acknowledging a point beyond which the current level and quality of services cannot possibly be retained if further reduction of health care costs is to be imposed.

Job Content

Reporting

The financial manager is expected to report appropriately on the financial activities and operations of the institution. Such reporting usually takes the form of monthly and annual financial statements. Income statements encompass the results from hospital operations on an ongoing basis. The balance sheet reflects the financial condition of the institution at a specific point in time. Monthly financial information will generally be compared to a budget on a month-to-month and year-to-year basis. Included are details that management and the governing board feel are appropriate under the circumstances. While financial operations may be measured against a budget and level of activity that was anticipated for the institution, the status of the balance sheet and its assets and liabilities must be measured against some other set of standards. Specific reports in this regard may compare against a base period set of ratios or measurements, such as those from the previous fiscal year-end balance sheet. Items to be included here could be such things as days of income outstanding in accounts receivable, days of expense outstanding in accounts payable, current ratio, or inventory turnover ratios.

Other management reports are also the responsibility of the financial manager. These include reports to departments on the status of their individual budgets, accounting for such items as the payroll dollars that are being expended, and the inventory withdrawals charged to the department. Such information needs to be communicated regularly to the individual department heads. The department head bears individual responsibility for departmental financial operations, and he or she obviously requires such regular reporting information.

The financial manager is also responsible for preparing reports to outside authorities such as federal, state, and local governments, as well as to cost-based third parties. Survey data including statistical or financial information for associations and government are prepared under the auspices of the financial manager. So is information relative to financing either on a short-term or long-term basis, and compliance reports to federal or state governments and their agencies, in order to fulfill Hill-Burton tax exemption, or fund raising requirements.

Accounting Services

For the purpose of explanation here the accounting services function has been divided into three parts: general accounting, payroll, and accounts payable. *General accounting* includes the recording of all the transactions of the institution, whether for services rendered, services and supplies acquired, or gifts received and expended. The general accounting department accounts for the day-to-day operations of the institution in terms of its general or unrestricted funds. This department processes information on the institution's restricted funds (those grants or gifts received to be used for a specified purpose), its endowment funds (those donated funds the principal of which is to be invested, and only the income to be used for a restricted or unrestricted purpose), agency funds (those funds held for others over which the institution provides only custodial services and does not control), and plant funds (land, building, fixed assets, and equipment acquisitions and liabilities of the institution).

The *payroll* function utilizes the data obtained at the time of hire and during subsequent promotion or increase periods to maintain an individual on the payroll records of the institution. Payroll systems within the health care institutions are particularly complex because of the significant variations in pay even for the same job. For example, different work shifts (day, middle, night, weekends, holidays, overtime) call for different pay. The payroll for any individual employee may vary from one week to the next. The fact that a hospital employee may work in two separate departments on two different jobs at two different rates of pay requires that a complex system maintain and control these payrolls.

The *accounts payable* department processes the payment of all nonsalaried expenditures, excluding perhaps expenditures associated with a major construction program. Unique purchase arrangements with certain vendors for special discounting arrangements or timely payment require constant monitoring.

Receivables Management

Since most health care institutions operate on a limited margin, the proper management of accounts receivable is essential for cash flow. An admitting and registration system, whether for inpatient or outpatient services, is indispensable. The admitting or registration department must collect appropriate data on newly admitted patients. This so-called front end work includes the collection of personal and financial data on individual patients.

Receivables management includes timely billing for services. An itemized bill for all services rendered is provided to the patient or the third-party payer responsible for the patient as soon after the patient's discharge as is possible. The billing process may be delayed by late charges, or billing may have to await approval of the patient's coverage by a third party.

Receivables management also includes collection of payments from self-pay patients who have failed to pay their bills in a timely fashion. Collection of delayed payments applies also to bills to delinquent third-party payers. Collection policies are established to determine whether the particular patient qualifies for free care or whether an account should be written off as a bad debt.

Cost Reimbursement, Rate Review, and Cost Accounting

These activities include filing appropriate reports for governmental or third-party reimbursement or the filing of rate requests with independent commissions or agencies set up to determine such rates. Medicare and Medicaid require that annual cost reports for each health care institution be filed within three months of the close of the fiscal or accounting year. Other third parties, such as Blue Cross, may have their own sets of cost reports requiring completion. Any filing for a rate adjustment or change must take place prior to the date of such change, and, in the case of a fiscal year, usually a few months prior to the beginning of that period.

Meticulous strategy is essential in the preparation of these reports or filings. The financial officer must analyze regulations and rules with care. This activity is analogous to the process used in the for profit industries in the filing of tax returns, wherein one properly takes advantage of all areas permitted within the tax regulations for the industry's maximum deduction and greatest recovery of cost. There is also long-term strategy within the institution. The type of reimbursement for specific services and the limitations on certain types of cost affect decisions to proceed with certain programs or activities and modify others.

The analysis of costs falls within this activity: to identify all costs and to analyze the impact of each cost on each activity. Cost-benefit analyses and analyses of return on investment have become reliable aids to decision making.

The financial manager must negotiate with third parties either directly or through a spokesman, such as the hospital association. Accordingly, he or she must have a thorough knowledge of the pertinent contracts, regulations, and processes, in order to judge what improvements are necessary both for the financial benefit of the institution as well as for practical ease of compliance.

Budgeting

The financial manager must help prepare the hospital's annual budget. Preparation requires extensive statistical forecasts in order to identify, particularly in a regulated environment, what is the extent of cost recognition or reimbursement. The manager then derives budgetary guidelines that identify limitations for certain cost increases. He or she must measure the availability of funds for capital expenditures early in the process of preparing the budget in order to help management evaluate alternatives and provide guidelines to departments for the level of reasonable expenditures to request.

Budgetary activity means periodically monitoring the costs of operation of the individual departments against their budgets during the year. Overruns in certain departments need early recognition in order to alert the departments to take remedial action. Today's sophisticated budget operation often includes a budgetary control function that operates on the premise that certain costs will not be incurred without a preapproval or clearance process.

Data Processing

Data processing has become a conventional feature in industrial administration, although its arrival in the health care industry occurred relatively late. The realization of its benefits did not come to full light until the 1970s. Because of the eventual application of data processing to many activities other than the strictly financial ones, there are recurrent pressures to transfer data processing from finance to elsewhere in the table of institutional organization. Such a shift in locus of activity would be a major mistake, in my view. Within any institution there should be one, or at the most two, areas where data processing operates. The first—and, obviously, the preferable one—is in the department of financial management, where most of the technical knowledge and control concepts exist. If data processing needs to stand alone in the future, it should function as an independent activity under strong data processing leadership that reports to the chief executive officer, and not to a subsidiary administrative officer. Development of the so-called data base for the institution could effectively provide information for use to all who require it. For example, patient data, rather than being maintained in the receivables department, the medical records department, and the ancillary services, could be collected in one place and shared by all through access to a single computerized data base.

Materiel Management

The increasingly important management of materiel in the health care field places under one function the request for, receipt of, distribution of, and disposal of all materiel utilized by the institution. Such a concentration of function maximizes the purchasing power, minimizes the storage costs, and makes for standardization and improved quality.

The materiel management function begins with acquisition of supplies and materials. Controlling quality and utilization of the materiel gives the financial manager an opportunity to maximize financial benefits for the institution. Storing supplies and goods according to type, monitoring their turnover, and identifying obsolescence of goods also helps to maximize financial benefits by minimizing duplication of materials and products.

Supply distribution today shows the greatest need for improvement. Regrettably, the manner in which many hospitals request, pick up, and transport supplies is inefficient. For example, sending nurses to a storeroom to pick up a handful of items on a regular basis is a misuse of personnel. A well-designed and business-oriented distribution system addressed to providing the appropriate quantities needed in different areas can produce substantial savings in the cost of personnel and storage of supplies.

Other areas are often categorized under materiel management: laundry and linen distribution, escort messsenger service, pharmacy, housekeeping, and so forth.

Internal Audit

The auditing approach is most often defined as the function which outside auditors or independent certified public accountants perform. Financial auditing as well as operational auditing, however, can be conducted by an internal audit department. Financial auditing performed by the internal audit function usually constitutes activities which the external auditors do not perform. Review of inventories, payroll distributions, or the effectiveness of reporting systems can be categorized as financial.

Operational auditing has been added to the responsibilities of the department as it evaluates financial and other activities within individual departments. Operational auditing scrutinizes the efficiency of the individual departments' activities and questions whether their actual use of resources is furthering their explicit objectives.

In some institutions the internal audit function may not report outside the financial management structure in order to preserve its independence.

Capital Financing

Assume that an institution ascertains that it needs major capital financing, or that it wishes to refinance existing indebtedness. The financial manager's initial involvement is to assess the institution's feasibility to carry the proposed indebtedness over future financial periods. To accomplish this, a significant amount of data must be collected and analyzed. The problems of forecasting and the formulation of projections in light of reimbursement changes make this an expensive and time-consuming process, often requiring the assistance of outside personnel.

The health care institution has various options for financing. These may change from one period to the next, depending on changes in state laws, reimbursement, federal regulatory policies, and the marketplace. In considering its options—tax-exempt bonds, federally subsidized or insured mortgages, its own indenture notes, commercial financing, or bank financing—the institution needs to evaluate the benefits and costs of each. Outside assistance may be necessary both for analyzing the marketplace and for determining cost effectiveness. The financial manager has much to say about the financing or refinancing vehicle.

Investments

Investments can be either short- or long-term. Short-term investments generally fall within the responsibility of the financial manager. These include the investment of short-term monies that await expenditure or are idle for a limited period of time. Endowment funds or capital expenditure funds for the future ordinarily are excluded.

Long-term investments are relatively permanent investments, such as endowment funds or long-term restricted funds. These are generally managed by an investment committee of the governing board, or perhaps by its finance committee. The financial manager's department will usually provide staff and reports for this activity.

Short-term investments include treasury bills, certificates of deposit, commercial paper, money market funds, daily investment funds, and, in some instances, Eurodollars and Yankee dollars. Long-term investments usually take the form of equity stocks or bonds which are generally balanced between yield return and growth potential. The philosophy for long-term investments will vary according to market conditions and the intention of the investment committee relative to the use of the funds.

Cash Management

The constraints on reimbursement, together with economic conditions, have increased the importance of cash management. The use of lock boxes and computerized tape-to-tape billing are obvious efforts to bring cash in more quickly. Other methods include (1) establishing bank accounts so that outstanding balances are invested for as long as possible and (2) making disbursements in such a way as to maximize the outstanding period. Maintaining a minimum of zero balance, thereby maximizing to the greatest extent possible the funds which may be invested on a short-term basis, requires daily monitoring by the financial manager.

Hospitals, like many businesses, require a line of credit that can be drawn upon when peak cash demands or lags in cash receipts occur. Managing the use of the line of credit in lieu of other dollars available to the institution, either from within or from outside, and maintaining the line relationship with the banks are the responsibilities of the financial manager.

Grants and Contracts

While applicable generally to larger teaching institutions, the financial aspects of grants and contracts with outside agencies or foundations also fall under the responsibility of the financial manager. Grants and contracts, particularly those received from the federal government, require precise accounting and monitoring. Funds specifically awarded must be used for their intended purpose and can be reallocated in only a very limited degree. Certain types of payment require government preapproval, whereas others can put the institution in technical violation of the federal government's guidelines. Intimate knowledge of all these requirements is essential in order to protect the institution from embarrassment and liability.

The degree of cost sharing that takes place is important to both the institution and the granting agency. Cost sharing refers to that portion of the research activities supported by funds not provided by the government. Identifying other sources of matching funds which will minimize the need for using hospital resources is preferable. The larger the research activity, the greater the potential for dollars to be saved or lost.

Government contracts and nongovernment contracts provide varying degrees of overhead recovery for those nondirect expenses applicable to the grant. Since certain grants do not pay the full overhead, whereas others pay overhead which need not be counted against overhead costs, the financial manager and the staff must be aware of the flexibilities of the overhead recovery process and how these apply to different activities. Accounting for such overhead costs in a more specific way may, at times, improve the total recovery that an institution can expect for grants.

Insurance

The traditional role for the financial manager has been the maintenance of insurance coverage for the institution. This involves the traditional property and liability insurance on its activities, as well as any other specialized coverage. In recent years, with the significant growth in the cost of malpractice insurance, institutions have begun to move into a program of risk management with the establishment of a risk manager. The maintenance of insurance coverage other than for malpractice continues to be the responsibility of the financial manager. Keeping up-to-date on the unique premium pricing mechanisms that have changed recently is necessary in order to assure the institution of the lowest cost for insurance.

Claims management is at times the responsibility of the financial manager or the staff. Usually the manager or someone else merely serves as the conduit for claims as they are forwarded to the appropriate insurance representatives.

Goals and Objectives

Modern planning in health care institutions calls particular attention to financial planning. The financial manager needs to have major input into this process and to keep the institution advised of the resources that may be available in the future. The impact of new programs that the institution may be planning requires analysis and projection by the financial manager's staff. Steps that need to be taken to maximize and maintain the financial well-being of the institution in the future fall within their purview.

Information

The financial manager is often the individual who is called upon by outside agencies to provide additional information on the finances or the reports which have been prepared by the institution. New legislation and new regulations will be referred to the financial manager for comments and recommendations. The financial manager must remain alert to all developments pertinent to his or her professional areas of concern.

Reporting Responsibilities

Management Level

Within the managerial table of organization the financial manager, as the number two or three person, participates in making major managerial decisions as well as providing information and consultation on financial matters.

Finance Committee

The financial manager communicates his or her views about current operations and financial strategy to the board through its finance committee, to which he or she acts as staff to provide pertinent documentation and analyses. The finance committee refers a summary of its findings and conclusions on financial matters to the full governing board. The financial manager and the staff translate financial policies adopted by the full board into financial programs.

Audit Committee

A separate audit committee of the governing board commonly exists in order to review the audit process, the audit report, and the auditor's management letter. This committee should maintain its independence from the finance committee, which is typically involved with the operations of the institution. The audit committee is more remote from such operations and thus performs a useful objective function. Attending audit committee meetings along with governing board members would be the financial manager, the external auditor, the internal auditor, and the chief executive or operating officer.

Governing Board

The financial manager also attends the meetings of the governing board, joining the chief executive officer and the chief operating officer. Although the finance committee may have completed an extensive review of the financial statements and related matters, board members often feel more comfortable directing their inquiries to the financial manager rather than to some intermediary. In some organizations financial matters are of sufficient gravity to require the financial manager to attend executive committee meetings of the board as well.

Institutional Uniqueness

Structural and organizational differences among institutions lead to idiosyncratic financial programs and policies. The financial needs and the demands of a community hospital obviously differ from those of a teaching hospital. The community hospital bears the inescapable responsibility to provide initial, basic services to patients within the hospital's catchment area. The teaching voluntary hospital provides more sophisticated tertiary care and generally bears higher costs.

As part of an overall educational institution, a university hospital lacks the independence of an individual hospital. Its unique relationships to the medical school have their own financial implications. Similar comments are in order for hospitals under the several types of governmental auspices, since type of clientele and method of payment will create a distinct set of financial variables.

New Developments

The imperatives of institutional survival, the drive toward more stringent economies, and the impetus toward regionalization will encourage more hospital mergers. At the same time, one may expect expansion of management companies that assume partial or complete administrative control of an institution or provide services to an institution at the senior administrative level. The financial manager has much to contribute to these new developments aimed primarily at greater financial efficiencies.

Autobiography

How does one become a financial manager in health administration? A look at my own career may be instructive. The fact that my father and my brother were accountants influenced me initially to decide on a career in public accounting. After obtaining a Bachelor of Science degree in accounting at Fordham University, I joined the New York City office of Haskins & Sells. The firm had a large staff and varied clients, including numerous brokerage houses and banks. For me, counting securities over a weekend and working on some unimaginative audit tasks were not too challenging, so I was happy to be selected to serve on the audit of the New York University, the nation's largest private educational institution. After several years on the N.Y.U. audit, I was assigned to some special work for the University's Medical Center that was serviced by a separate audit team.

I became fascinated with the nonprofit sector. My interests transcended accounting and auditing problems and encompassed management as well. In 1966 I accepted a standing invitation to join the staff of the New York University Medical Center as manager of cost accounting, a new department at the medical center. Although the experience there proved to be extensive, the opportunity for me to move further into the financial management structure did not materialize as I had expected.

In 1968 I accepted the post of Assistant Director of Financial Affairs at two hospitals in Philadelphia—Misericordia Hospital and Fitzgerald-Mercy Hospital. I participated in planning and implementing the merger of the two 400-bed hospitals owned by the same religious order into one fiscal and legal entity. Following completion of the merger in 1969, I became the Chief Financial Officer of the new institution. In 1972 a physician president of one of the major area hospitals urged me to join the staff as Executive Vice-President, effectively promoting me to the position of the hospital administrator. I agreed, but with the proviso that I give the job a two-year trial period to ascertain whether I liked the role of administrator. During this time I was heavily involved professionally in the local chapter of the Hospital Financial Management Association and nationally as the association's lecturer on cost containment. In 1974, at the end of the two years, I decided that I preferred financial management, and accepted a position as Associate Director for Fiscal Affairs at the Peter Bent Brigham Hospital in Boston, Massachusetts.

The hospital, Harvard Medical School's primary teaching affiliate, had been encountering financial difficulties, and, by January of 1975, it was to merge with two other hospitals, the Boston Hospital for Women and the Robert B. Brigham Hospital. Over the succeeding years the financial departments of all the institutions were merged, financial management was centralized, and a new facility was financed and constructed. The *de facto* merger took longer to accomplish, with the merger of most medical departments not occurring until just before the physical movement into the new facility in mid-1980.

In 1979, I was invited to return to public accounting as a partner with an international C.P.A. firm. I decided to defer such a move until I had completed all my objectives at the merged Affiliated Hospitals Center. In 1980 the same firm came back to me with an additional offer to concentrate exclusively on health care. On July 1, 1980, I joined Touche, Ross & Co. in Boston as an audit partner with ongoing responsibility for hospital clients. I am now on the firm's national service committee for health care, deciding policy and practice for the firm's services in the health care field.

I have thus made a complete career circle, from public accounting to the hospital field and back into public accounting with concentration on hospital affairs, without having specifically planned it that way.

Every would-be financial manager in health administration will doubtless pursue a different path, but will find at last two things in common: formal education and experience in finance and in health administration.

17 Health Services Administration in the Canadian Context

John M. Phin, M.D., and Edwin Chown

The similarities between Canada and the United States sometimes obscure the palpable differences between the two governments, and the diverse histories and cultures of the two friendly nations. How these differences affect the careers of health administrators is discussed in the following chapter by John M. Phin, M.D., and Edwin Chown. (L.E.B.)

At the broad conceptual level, health services administrators throughout the world engage in similar activities. Health administration has been defined as "planning, organizing, directing, controlling, and coordinating the resources and procedures by which needs and demands for health and medical care and a healthful environment are fulfilled by the provision of specific services to individual clients, organizations and communities."[1] In practice, the way in which an administrator of health services undertakes this task is influenced to a great extent by the characteristics of the country and region where he or she works.

Canadians have much in common with their neighbors to the south. Indeed, the many similarities at times tend to overshadow the significant differences in the political, social, economic, and cultural contexts of the two countries. Although an in-depth discussion of these differences is beyond the scope of this article, it is important to acknowledge that health administrators in Canada work in an environment different from that of their American counterparts. This may not be apparent to the casual observer. However, the origins of the two countries, their dissimilar development, their different forms of government, and their differing approaches to social legislation and social policy development require more study than can be provided here.[2]

Historical Perspective

The existence of a comprehensive "national" health insurance system in Canada has a major influence on the nature and shape of the health delivery system.[3] Hospital services were insured following federal legislation in 1958. Ten years later medical services were insured with the passage of a similar act. In both cases, the federal acts were essentially funding mechanisms to provide money to the provinces if they instituted insurance programs which met certain broad, basic criteria. All provinces opted into the programs to take advantage of the cost-sharing formula. In the late 1970s, a transfer of tax points and other similar mechanisms were introduced to replace the cost-sharing approach, providing the provinces with greater flexibility in the expenditure of health dollars.

Programs of health insurance were in operation in Canada long before the federal legislation in 1958. During the 1920s and 1930s, smaller communities in western Canada recognized the importance of health care and worked through municipal governments to recruit and pay physicians. Similar programs for hospital care, known as

John M. Phin, M.D., is Executive Director of the Canadian College of Health Service Executives; Edwin Chown is Director of Education, Canadian Hospital Association.

union hospital districts, were also developed. These pioneering schemes of health insurance led to proposals for provincial plans in most of the provinces, particularly during the Depression years when the costs of health care were disastrous for the many unemployed. Saskatchewan was the first province to introduce both hospital and medical insurance (in 1947 and 1962 respectively). The success of insurance in that province was one of the factors leading to the development of the federal legislation.

Now the provincial governments are the source of over 88 percent of all health care expenditures.[4] As a consequence, major policy decisions tend to be made at the provincial level, and there is increasing emphasis on regional planning of services. As Canadians have tended to look to various levels of government to finance and coordinate the provision of health services, most health programs are now heavily influenced by governmental legislation and regulation with only a few elements (such as drugs) being provided in a competitive marketplace. Health services in Canada are viewed as a system, made up of components intended to function in concert with the rest of the system to serve the public good.

Although health services are provided under the umbrella of an insurance program, this system does not operate with complete harmony and bliss. Many decisions require discussion and debate among representatives of the parts of the system and also by politicians and the public. For example, how much should be spent on health care? How should such expenditure be allocated among sectors of the health system and among individual institutions and programs? What is quality? The resolution of these issues requires knowledgeable and skilled leadership.

Career Paths in Canada

The professional health administrator with broad orientation to the total health system can be a central force in facilitating policy decisions. Where in the past an administrator in one of the various sectors of health care (for example, hospitals, nursing homes, mental health programs) tended to act in isolation within his or her own sector (to the possible detriment of the patient or client who is often using more than one of the sectors), increasingly younger and better educated health executives see their role as an intermediary between sectors. Where once an administrator failed to see movement in his or her career between sectors as a benefit to career development, the health executive now views such movement positively. In brief, the health executive views the health services as an interrelated system providing opportunities to exercise management skills in many parts of the system. The career development of many administrators may include movement through health management positions in provincial governments (Ministries of Health, Ministries of Social Services, regional health councils, or provincial or regional public health units). This is a more usual and more acceptable career path than for their U.S. counterparts, and one which then influences future behavior. The health executive who has been for part of his or her career a part of the government bureaucracy dealing with a broader than local perspective of the health service is likely to see government involvement and intervention in health services in a different light than one whose experience has been limited to a specific institution or series of local facilities.

The estimated 8,000 health services executives in Canada are employed by the following agencies: acute care institutions, long-term care facilities, federal government, provincial governments, public health units, district/regional planning councils, health associations, consulting firms, home care agencies, group clinics, and the armed forces.

If there is anything unique about Canadian health services administration career development, it is this systems orientation. While most executives tend to develop careers within one of these sectors, there is increasing movement between sectors. In part, such moves are motivated by an individual's desire to develop greater knowledge of the health system. But this flexibility of career path is also a reflection of the

Canadian educational programs in health administration which have tended to be less specialized than those in the United States.

Education in Health Administration in Canada

Graduate programs in health administration developed in a similar fashion to those in the United States. The first program was started in 1947 with a hospital focus. Over the years four others were established and now all have a broad health services perspective (although there are some differences in emphasis among programs). These programs require two years of study on a full-time basis, and several allow for part-time study. Three of the five also provide doctoral programs with an emphasis in health administration.

The development of graduate education in health services administration in Canada was paralleled by noncredit extension courses of two years' duration for practicing health care managers. These courses are sponsored by the Canadian Hospital Association and some universities. These courses provide mid-career educational opportunities primarily for senior health managers who lack specialized preparation and also for middle managers who want to improve their knowledge and skills in health services administration. Most of the students in these courses have specialized clinical or technical training but have moved into management positions in mid-career. The extension format has allowed managers from any community to enroll.

Most recently baccalaureate level programs have emerged at four universities. In Canada, these all are part-time mid-career degree programs for practicing managers in health organizations. The delivery formats are varied. As mentioned in chapter 1, there are no programs of accreditation for undergraduate education. Consequently potential students should examine baccalaureate programs with care to determine their scope and depth and their reputation in the field. Optimally, the applicant should determine his or her own objectives and then determine the program which can best assist in the meeting of these.

Almost all Canadian university programs participate actively in the Association of University Programs in Health Administration (AUPHA). In addition, graduate level programs are accredited by the Accrediting Commission on Education for Health Services Administration.

Once an individual has entered the field of practice in health administration in Canada, he or she is eligible to join the field's professional organization, the Canadian College of Health Service Executives. This association enrolls executives from all sectors of the health system and is devoted to their ongoing professional development. By bringing senior managers together, the College reinforces the broad systems approach to health services in Canada.

NOTES

[1]Charles J. Austin, "What Is Health Administration?" *Hospital Administration* 19, 3 (Summer 1974):p. 27.

[2]For a thorough analysis of the Canadian health care environment, see the anthology *Perspectives on Canadian Health and Social Services Policy: History and Emerging Trends*, Carl A. Meilicke, Ph.D., and Janet L. Storch, M.H.S.A., eds. Ann Arbor, Michigan: Health Administration Press, 1980.

[3]For a full description and analysis of the development of health insurance in Canada, see Malcolm G. Taylor, *Health Insurance and Canadian Public Policy: The Seven Decisions That Created the Canadian Health Insurance System.* Montreal: McGill-Queens University Press, 1978.

[4]*National Health Expenditures 1969–1973.* Ottawa, Canada: Health Economics and Statistics, Health Programs Branch, Health and Welfare, April 1976.

Reference
Supplement

This Reference Supplement consists of a list of major organizations which are sources of information for health services administration education and practice. The referenced practitioner organizations collectively reflect the many practice areas staffed by health administrators. More information about career pathways and education opportunities can be gained if this Supplement is used as a starting point in the quest for specific details and general literature.

Information Sources

Accrediting Commission on Education for Health Services Administration
One Dupont Circle, Suite 420
Washington, D.C. 20036   (202) 659-3939

American Academy of Medical Administrators
2590 E. Devon Avenue, Suite 107
Des Plaines, Illinois 60018   (312) 827-5890

American Association of Hospital Consultants
2341 Jefferson Davis Highway
Arlington, Virginia 22202   (703) 528-2700

American College of Hospital Administrators
840 North Lake Shore Drive
Chicago, Illinois 60611   (312) 943-0544

American College of Medical Group Administrators
4101 E. Louisiana Avenue
Denver, Colorado 80222   (303) 753-1111

American College of Nursing Home Administrators
4650 East-West Highway
Washington, D.C. 20014   (202) 652-8384

American Health Planning Association
1601 Connecticut Avenue, N.W., Suite 700
Washington, D.C. 20009   (202) 232-6390

American Hospital Association
840 North Lake Shore Drive
Chicago, Illinois 60611   (312) 280-6000

American Public Health Association
1015 15th Street, N.W.
Washington D.C. 20005   (202) 789-5600

Association of Mental Health Administrators
425 13th Street, N.W., Suite 1230
Washington, D.C. 20004   (202) 638-6662

Association of University Programs in Health Administration
One Dupont Circle, Suite 420
Washington, D.C. 20036   (202) 659-4354

Canadian College of Health Service Executives
410 Laurier Avenue West, Suite 805
Ottawa, Ontario K1R 7T3   (613) 235-7218

Canadian Hospital Association
410 Laurier Avenue, West, Suite 800
Ottawa, Ontario K1R 7T6   (613) 238-8005

Canadian Public Health Association
1335 Carling Avenue, Suite 306
Ottawa, Ontario K1Z 8N8   (613) 725-3769

Federation of American Hospitals, Inc.
1111 19th Street, N.W., Suite 402
Washington, D.C. 20036   (202) 833-3090

Hospital Financial Management Association
1900 Spring Road, Suite 500
Oak Brook, Illinois 60521   (312) 655-4600

Medical Group Management Association
4101 E. Louisiana Avenue
Denver, Colorado 80222   (303) 753-1111

National Association of Health Services Executives
2231 S. Western Avenue
Los Angeles, California 90018   (213) 737-7372

NOTES

NOTES

NOTES

NOTES

NOTES

NOTES

NOTES

NOTES